Nicki Waterman's

Flat
Stomach
Plan

Nicki Waterman's

Flat Stomach Plan

The Ultimate Abdominal Workouts and Diet

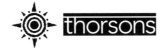

Thorsons
An Imprint of HarperCollins*Publishers*
77–85 Fulham Palace Road
Hammersmith, London W6 8JB

The website address is:
www.thorsonselement.com

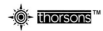

and *Thorsons* are trademarks of
HarperCollins*Publishers* Limited

First published by Thorsons 2003

10 9 8 7 6 5 4 3 2 1

All clothes worn by Nicki have been designed by
HOMMEBODY – 'A Lifestyle Collection for Women
on the Move'

A catalogue record of this book
is available from the British Library

ISBN 0 00 714373 7

Photographs © Guy Hearn

Printed and bound in Great Britain by
Martins the Printers Limited, Berwick upon Tweed

Contents

Introduction

So you want to have a nice flat tum? Well who doesn't? If you want to look in the mirror and see a tummy you would be proud to show, then the best way of going about it is to do the 'curl'.

Of course, curls on their own aren't a magic bullet to a wonderful new you. A firm tummy buried beneath a thick layer of fat will still protrude and look flabby. If you do the curl three or four times a week and don't tackle the problem by any other means then, yes, you will still tone up your tummy (as well as improve your posture and help prevent backache). However, to really flatten your stomach and see the pounds drop off you need to take three steps:

1. Do the curl three or four times a week.
2. Do an aerobic workout every day.
3. Eat sensibly.

If you combine a regular abs session with healthy eating and an overall workout programme that includes aerobic activity, then not only will those pounds drop off, but your body shape will be transformed.

What is the curl?

So what exactly is the curl and why will it work for you? In simple terms, the curl is an exercise that tones up the abdomen by tightening and then relaxing the network of muscles of the stomach and waist – muscles known as the abdominals, or abs. And the stronger the abs, the flatter the stomach.

The most effective way of toning up the abs is to shorten the distance between your ribcage and your pelvis by repeatedly contracting the muscles in your abdomen. Sports science has shown that the best and safest way of achieving this is by using your stomach muscles to lift your upper back off the floor towards your middle (curl) and to lift the hips and bring them up towards your chest (reverse curl). The best method of defining the waist is to subject the abdominal muscles that run around the midriff to twists.

Achieving a flat, strong stomach may be your goal for the simple reason that it looks good, but it is desirable for other reasons too. Well-trained abs help to prevent lower back pain, as well as encouraging good posture, a well-aligned body and a general sense of well-being.

Like all the best modern workout programmes, abs training has a lot of sports science behind it. It is carefully devised, well thought-out and safe. And, as I pointed out before, the curl – or 'the crunch' as it is also known – is recognized as one of the most effective forms of ab training.

So how does ab training work?

Let's start with a quick anatomy lesson so that you understand what is going on inside you. The pelvic girdle – the ring of bone that your legs are connected to – is the bowl in which many of your vital organs sit. To keep them in there and to protect them from harm, you need more than your pelvis, backbone and your skin – you need a firm wall of abdominal muscles. These muscles also give you the ability to bend forward and to twist from the waist. (At the back of the body are the back muscles, which, together with your backbone and ribcage, help support your frame and hold you upright. I look at these in more detail in Chapter 8.)

Your abdominal muscles consist of a thick layer – a sheet almost – of overlapping fibres that stretch downwards from your ribcage to your pelvis and wrap sideways around you from your spine to the front of your pelvis, like the interlocking fingers of both hands.

The main muscle is the rectus abdominus, which stretches vertically from the ribs (directly beneath your breasts) to the front of the pelvic girdle. The oblique abdominals start at your spine and wrap, in a forward and downward slant, around your body in two layers (internal and external) to the pelvic girdle. Finally there are the transverse abs, which fan out from the ribs to the pelvis across your lower abdomen.

Forward flexion – bending down

You are able to bend from the waist thanks to the action of the rectus abdominus. This is a very strong and long muscle that appears to be divided in two down a line running between your sternum and navel. In fact, it is one big muscle joined by thin sheets of muscle fibre. (It can, however, separate along this 'join' during pregnancy – see page 98.) This is the muscle that is strengthened and toned during forward curls.

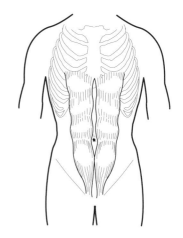

Rotation and forward flexion – bending and twisting

The internal and external obliques not only ensure that we can rotate our torso (for example to turn sideways when driving so we can look behind us) but they also assist in forward flexion. A nice bonus of well-toned obliques is that your waist gets slimmer and more defined. We strengthen and tone these muscles by adding a twist to the basic curl. (Note: whenever you work one side, you should always work the opposite side.)

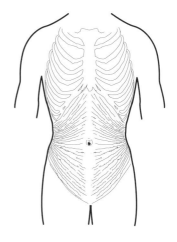

The breathing powerhouse

The transverse abs, which fan out from the middle across the lower half of your abdomen to the sides of your pelvic girdle, do the most work in protecting your internal organs. At the same time, they assist in breathing. The diaphragm is known as the bellows of the lungs, but if you take a deep breath and then exhale you will be able to feel the transverse abs helping to expel the air. It is these muscles that work hard in a basic curl and that make the lower half of your tummy flat.

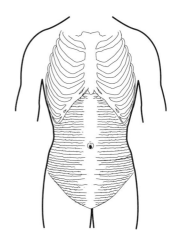

Curls vs sit-ups

It was once widely thought – and still is amongst a few trainers who aren't all that well-informed or up to date – that sits-ups were the ideal means of strengthening the abs. Undoubtedly, sit-ups do have a role in advanced sports training – but they are not the most efficient or effective way of working the abs or getting a flat tummy.

Research has shown that sit-ups use the hip flexor muscles (at the back of the thighs) and the quadriceps, or quads (at the front of the thighs), more than the abdominals. This is because the abdominal muscles are only used to start the sit-up (the first 30–45 degrees). In addition, since the hip flexors are attached from the thigh to the lower spine, a sit-up exaggerates the natural curve of the spine thereby increasing the risk of injury in that area. Hence, doing too many sit-ups or doing them incorrectly can put too great a strain on the back and the stomach muscles, leading to injury.

There is no doubt – and science has proved it – the curl is a far safer and more effective way of strengthening and flattening your stomach.

Some myths about abs training

Before we move on to the practicalities of using this book, there are a few misunderstandings about abs training that I must dispel upfront.

Curls will give you a flat stomach

Yes, they will – but not on their own. Sadly, you can't spot reduce fat. When you lose weight, the fat is taken from all parts of the body equally. Specific exercises tone up and de-flab the targeted area, but if that area is hidden beneath a thick layer of fat, no amount of exercise in the world will make it look all that much flatter. You will get stronger muscles and a better posture, which are worthwhile achievements, but only ab training *combined* with a sensible eating programme will ultimately lead to a flat stomach that you can see.

Curls burn calories fast

Curls are not a high calorie burner. Yes, ab training does take a great deal of effort and effort does burn calories – but the key to a good ab session is slow and steady, not fast and furious. Ab training is the most effective way of toning up your abdominal muscles, but aerobic workouts raise the metabolism and therefore burn fat more efficiently. So ideally, if you want to lose your fat and flabby tum, you need to combine regular ab training with aerobic exercise and a sensible diet.

You need to do ab training every day for quick results

You should never work the same group of muscles day after day and certainly not on two consecutive days. This is because muscles develop during rest. When you train, muscle tissue is broken down. It then recuperates and strengthens during the following 48 hours – *if* it is allowed to rest.

It is best to put your hands behind your head during a curl

This isn't always necessary. When you are told to put your hands behind your head, it is for support. However, when you're a beginner and still struggling, the natural reflex action is to pull on your neck muscles as you come up. To prevent this, never clasp your fingers together – your hands should be open, your fingertips splayed and not touching and your head just resting in them for balance and support. Practise the correct position until you get it right. In many exercises you are asked not to put your hands behind your head – for example, sometimes it is recommended that you place your forearms alongside your ears for balance. Some trainers will suggest that it is best to put your hands on your chest or your fists at your ears. All you need to remember is to not pull on your head and neck when lifting. Let the contraction of your abs bring you up smoothly.

The upper and lower abs are two separate groups of muscles

The abdominals are one long sheet of interlocking muscle fibres. If an exercise says it works the upper or the lower abs, it simply means it works that area of the abdomen more. Curls target the upper abdominal area by bringing the upper back towards the pelvis. Reverse curls target the lower abdominal area by bringing the pelvis (hips) up towards the chest.

Is the curl safe?

In a nutshell – yes. But, as with all forms of exercise, seek the advice of your doctor, especially if you have an existing medical condition or orthopaedic limitations, such as a bad back or hip problems. You should always ask your doctor's advice if you are pregnant.

There are, in fact, very few people who are unable to do the curl and it is one of the few exercises that most people can do safely – whatever their age. Whether you're a teenager or an 80 year old, you'll find the curl can flatten your stomach, improve your posture, strengthen your back and curve in your waist.

How to Use this Book

First, read it. That may sound obvious, but that is exactly what you should do. Too often people just flick straight to the first exercise and get started without understanding what they are doing, or why they are doing it – and if you don't understand this it's very easy to do it wrong.

The exercise section of the book is designed in careful stages to take you through an entire abdominal workout programme from being a novice to becoming an expert. The core of the exercise section consists of four stages of development (see chapters 2–5), each of which you should complete and be comfortable with before moving on to the next. For the experienced, I have also included some very challenging curls and a total three-in-one routine (see pages 65–74).

There is an important chapter on preventing back problems, which includes back-strengthening exercises and specific cool-down techniques for the back. Additional chapters include ab training during and after pregnancy, and belly dancing – which I thoroughly endorse as a good form of aerobics combined with abdominal training. There is also a Curl-Free Workout, which is useful for challenging your ab muscles to do something a bit different.

The diet section of the book looks at healthy eating, and provides practical suggestions for delicious meals that are low in calories and fat. As I pointed out in the introduction, you can work hard to achieve a toned tum, but if it's hidden under a layer of fat you will not get that flat look you are aiming for. However, short-term, very restrictive diets are not the answer. In order to lose fat and keep it off, you need to adopt a healthy diet – the last two chapters show you how. The recipes are healthy and simple and provide an illustration of how easy it is for a sensible diet to become part of your everyday routine. And, of course, if healthy eating and exercise become second nature, you'll have that flat stomach for life.

Now before you're tempted to just dive in and get started, let's look at some of the practicalities of exercising those abs.

Warming up and cooling down

As always when working out, you should start your session by warming up and finish it by cooling down. Warming up is a kind of rehearsal for the actual exercises you will be doing. It raises your body temperature to ensure good circulation of blood and serves to lightly stretch the muscles you will be working, making them supple enough to prevent injury and minimize soreness. Cooling down eases everything back into place and relaxes you. Sections on warming up and cooling down for general ab training, as well as for back training, are included to teach you the correct techniques for each.

The four main abdominal training plans are as follows:

- Stage 1 is for beginners. It shows you all you will need to know and do to start a basic ab programme.
- Stage 2 is intermediate and focuses on increasing your strength. More areas of your abdominal muscles are brought into play as different and more complex techniques are introduced.
- Stage 3 is for the more experienced and focuses on 'shocking' the muscles by introducing more challenges in tempo, endurance and position, all of which encourage progress to new levels of fitness.
- Stage 4 is as demanding as it gets. Not to be undertaken by the inexperienced or unfit, this is your ultimate goal and when you have reached it you will have a truly awesome figure.

When you are ready

Before you begin your first workout, familiarize yourself with Chapter 2, Stage 1: Beginner's Curls. In this section, you will find advice and directions on how to breathe (it's not as simple as it sounds) and how to do a basic curl. It also illustrates how to position your body for the best effect and to avoid injury. Read, absorb and understand. When you have absorbed all this on paper, you will be ready to start. But don't proceed yet. First, comes the warm up. Before you do

Nicki Waterman's Flat Stomach Plan

anything else, you should always warm up. Chapter 1 is devoted to warm-up stretches specifically designed for your abdominal workout, so this is where your routine should always begin.

Now that you are ready to start, take it slowly – don't try to run before you can walk. Work your way through each stage, never moving on until you are completely confident and strong enough for each new and tougher challenge. If you have moved on too fast, stop, go back to the previous stage and do it all over again. It's quality not speed that counts in abs training. Your abdominal muscles will still get stronger and your stomach flatter, even if you always stay at Stage 1.

This is a good place to mention that if you have reached Stage 4 and need to stop for any length of time, it is advisable not to just throw yourself back in at the deep end when you start again. I strongly recommend that you start over with Stage 1 and work your way forward as a refresher. In fact, even if you are a Stage 4 super ab demon, it's good for your muscles to do a variety of exercises, so return to the exercises in the earlier stages now and again.

As you read all the various sections of this book, you will note that many of the warm up and cool-down exercises are similar and are repeated in full. This is to make using this book easier, so you don't have to keep flicking back and forth between sections.

Questions and answers

How often should I curl?

For maximum benefit, you need to exercise your abs three to four days a week, but not on consecutive days. Leave at least a day between each session (so, Monday, Wednesday, Friday, Sunday, Tuesday, Thursday and so on). As I've already explained, your muscles need time to recover.

How long should I work my abs?

Not less than 10 minutes. If that is all the time you can spare, it's still worth it. Beginners should train until they feel tired and then stop. Each exercise gives guidelines as to how many repetitions (reps) you should do, starting with about four and gradually increasing as you get stronger. Fifteen minutes overall is about right, especially if you are going to include abs training in with a workout plan that works all the muscles in your body. The main thing is never to strain or to keep on going if you are in pain.

What is the best time to do the curl?
Any time that you can set aside to exercise will do. However, I always suggest that early morning, as soon as you rise, is best because the rest of the day can get very crowded, especially if you lead a busy life. It's all too easy to tell yourself, 'I'll do it tomorrow' and often tomorrow ends up stretching into a week or a month of tomorrows and you just give up. If you really have no time, get up half an hour earlier. Exercise should be a regular part of your day.

How long will it take to get a flat stomach?
Provided that you're not huge to start with, you should see good results in as little as a week. In a month you will see a big improvement and in three months you should look and feel magnificent. If you're eating sensibly and doing aerobic exercise as well, you'll see results faster. Really, it's up to you and your determination.

> *Remember, you are in control of your body – not anyone else.*

Do I need to warm up for abs training if I have already warmed up for my other exercises?
Ideally, yes – because all warm-up stretches are designed for particular muscle groups. It is advisable to start every complete workout session with five or ten minutes of light aerobics – such as a brisk walk, dancing or running on the spot.

What about cooling down?
The same applies as above. Cooling down eases and relaxes those hard-worked and stretched muscles and helps prevent cramp.

You mention the back often. What's my back got to do with it – I thought ab training was for my abdominals?
Your back and abdominal muscles work together to give your torso a full range of movement. Weak stomach muscles often lead to back problems. Equally, there's

no point in over-training your front if you ignore your back. A strong, healthy body should have muscles that are worked equally all over as part of a total workout programme. I always suggest some back-strengthening exercises immediately after your abs cool down to keep the back muscles strong and supple (see Chapter 8). Remember to finish off with your back cool-down stretches.

You also mention good posture – why is this important?

Good posture not only looks good, it also means you're less likely to get back problems, your neck won't ache, you won't tire so easily and you will ease or even cure digestion and breathing problems. If you stand and sit correctly all your organs will be in their correct place, your muscles properly aligned and working correctly and, in turn, there won't be any strain on your joints. Good posture depends on having strong back and abdominal muscles. Together, they keep you upright and nicely in balance.

Do I really need to learn how to stand, sit and walk?

You shouldn't – after all, have you ever seen a young child with bad posture? However, as we get older many of us develop terrible posture. We stand for long hours with our weight balanced on one hip and knee, our spine twisted. We sit slumped in a chair, back curved, watching TV. We sit in car seats that are badly designed and put a huge strain on our middle and lower back. We sit at our desks all day, shoulders slumped forward, spine curved and stomach sagging. We even sleep on sagging mattresses with our backs bent and our necks twisted upwards on piles of pillows.

Well, how should I stand or sit then?

Stand with your feet hip-distance apart, your weight equally distributed, knees slightly relaxed and not pushed back and stiff. Your lower back should not be excessively arched in either a backward or forward direction. Try not to stand for long periods wearing high heels. Your shoulders should be back and down (not rounded forward or pulled back hard as if you've just joined the army). Your head, which is heavy, should be in the centre of your shoulders, not jutting forward. Your chin should be level, not up in the air. (Try it up – and feel the strain on the bones at the back of your neck. Now pull it far down and feel the strain on the muscles at the back of your neck.) Your neck has a natural curve that is designed to hold your head in the correct position. This is the basic position referred to throughout the curl exercises in this book.

Sit upright, back supported where possible, feet either flat on the floor in front of you or tucked back and balanced on the balls. Your stomach should be tucked in, buttocks against the back of the chair or a wall, hands resting lightly on thighs. If you have no back support, remember the Victorians. They used their muscles to hold them in an upright position – one thing they didn't do was slump or slouch.

So many people today shuffle around as if they are worn out, their head, belly and shoulders all aiming towards the ground, their backs rounded. They look as if they lack energy and drive – and it's not surprising.

Learn to stand and sit correctly and you will be amazed at the change, not only in your appearance but also in your attitude and motivation. You will dis-cover energy you never knew you had. And ab training really helps by first of all strengthening all the muscles that help keep your body upright and properly aligned. Add some back training and you will immediately notice a remarkable difference.

The illustrations opposite show how you should sit and stand.

Nicki Waterman's Flat Stomach Plan

Good Posture

Bad Posture

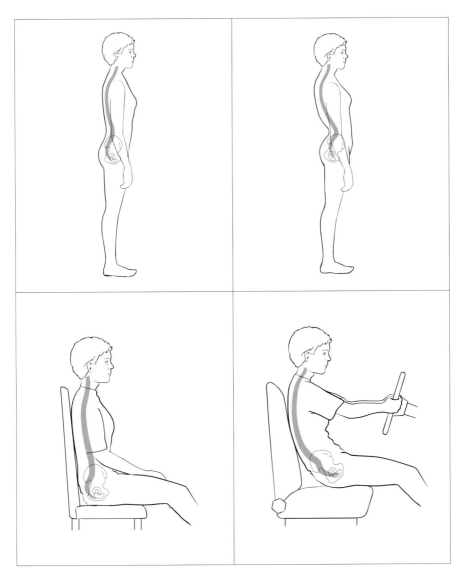

CHAPTER ONE

Warming Up

The purpose of warming up is self-explanatory: it is to make the body ready for exercise by raising the body temperature (and that of the joints and muscles, which will help prevent injury) and to promote good aerobic circulation. First you need to do some mild aerobic exercise to oxygenate the blood, to get the circulation going and to speed up your metabolism – brisk walking or running on the spot are both very effective.

You should never stretch cold. If your curl programme is not part of an overall exercise session working other muscles, or starts your workout, you should first do some mild aerobics, as described above, for about five minutes before stretching.

After your mild aerobic warm-up, it will be beneficial to spend just a few minutes sitting cross-legged on the floor, hands gently resting on your thighs, back straight, eyes focused straight ahead while you concentrate on some deep breathing and relaxing your muscles. Don't go into a meditative state – you need to keep your energy up – and don't stay there too long or you will cool down.

Now you're ready to stretch. Stretching is the best overall way of preparing the body for curls. It makes for greater overall flexibility, avoids damaging the muscles you will be working, reduces muscle tension, helps the circulation and clears the mind so that you are able to concentrate on your body and breathing.

Stretching should be slow and steady and never forced. Each stretch should be held for a maximum of ten counts since extreme flexibility is not what is required.

If you find any particular area is still stiff after the warm up, then repeat the warm-up exercise for that area

Sideways Neck Relax

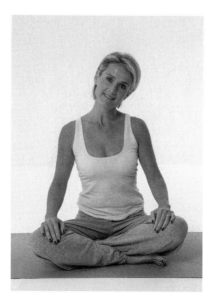

The purpose of this stretch is to relax the neck muscles so that they don't tense up during your curl programme. This is important since the neck can suffer strain during a lift – either because you are still inexperienced and pull on it with your hands, or because the muscles are not strong enough yet to fully support the weight of your head during some of the unsupported lifts. For this reason it is vital to always treat your neck with consideration and to get your posture right during the exercises.

Begin

You will already be seated cross-legged on the floor in the correct position for this if you have gone through your short preparation stage (see page 1). Make sure that your shoulders are down and relaxed and your abdomen lifted.

Next

Lower your head gently to your left shoulder, keeping the shoulders firmly down. Now bring your head smoothly up and lower to the right shoulder.

Do this 8–10 times on each side, avoiding jerky movements.

The Shoulder Shrug

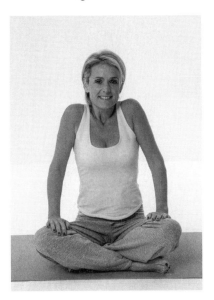

This stretch has the multiple effect of loosening the shoulders, neck and upper back.

Begin

Sit cross-legged on the floor with your back straight, your abs tucked in and up and your shoulders back. Let your arms hang down and forward, with your hands loosely hanging over your knees.

Next

Shrug both your shoulders up towards your ears. Hold. Release and repeat. To vary this a little as you release the shrug, try rolling your shoulders back and down.
Repeat 8–10 times.

Shoulder Back Pull

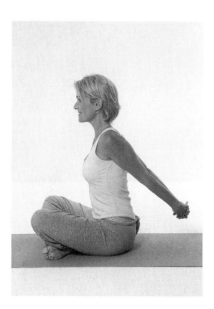

During curl exercises there is always a temptation to round your shoulders up and forwards to help with the lift, instead of relying solely on your abs. To counteract this we tend to put the shoulders under some degree of strain to keep down and back where they should be, so it is important to stretch and loosen the muscles across the front of your shoulders in readiness.

Begin
Sit upright, nice and straight, tummy tucked in and flat, your legs crossed loosely and with your arms low behind your buttocks, your hands clasped and loosely resting on the floor. Already you should feel your shoulders stretching and your chest expanding.

Next
Still maintaining your nice upright posture, lift your hands up and away from you as far as they will reach until you feel some tension in your shoulders. Keeping the arms straight, hold until you feel some easing of the tension, then raise them a little more to another degree of tension. Hold. The pattern should be tension and ease, tension and ease. Hold to a count of 8–10 and relax.

Nicki Waterman's Flat Stomach Plan

Bowing Forward

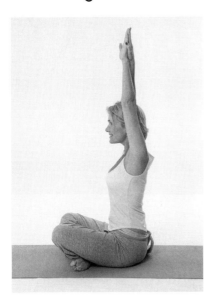 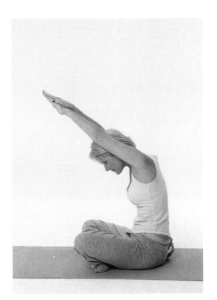

Now let's work your back muscles by doing a sleek, well-rounded curl.

Begin
Sit up nice and tall on the floor in a loose, cross-legged position and raise your arms straight above your head, palms forward and hands loosely lying in one another.

Next
Pull your tummy in and up as you curl forward as if bowing. Your arms should remain in the same position over your head – your upper body should move as a single unit. You should feel your back muscles stretching. Hold for a count of 8–10 then slowly lift back up to an upright position.

Lunge Stretch

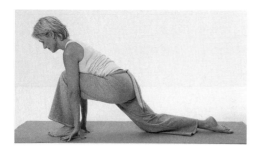

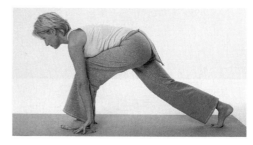

Begin

Kneel down on the floor. Now, ensuring that your head, neck and shoulders are all aligned correctly with your back – step forward and lean over your left knee. Your chest must remain lifted – don't sag in the middle or allow your head to droop. Your arms will be straight on either side of your left foot, fingertips resting on the floor.

Next

Holding your torso up, lunge forward slowly onto your left (front) leg, ensuring that the knee remains directly above the ankle. You should feel the front thigh muscles of the right (rear) leg stretch. Hold then relax.

Repeat on the other side.

Stand Up and Curl

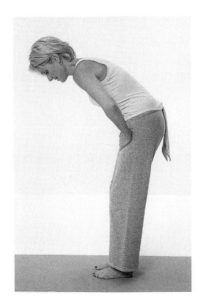

This is a good exercise for stretching the back.

Begin

Stand upright, legs hip-width apart and your hands on top of your thighs. Now lean over slightly from the hips, bending the knees a little – but don't sag. Make sure that your head, neck, shoulders and back are all aligned and your chest is lifted.

Next

Pull your tummy in as far as you can while continuing to keep your chest up and your head and back correctly aligned. You should feel the stretch in your back. Hold then relax.

Hip Circles

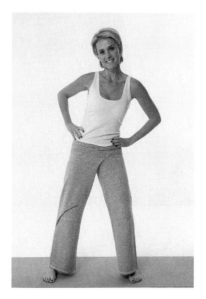 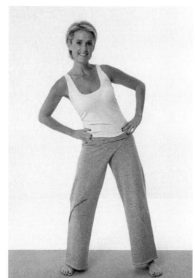

This exercise loosens up your hips and lower back.

Begin

Stand upright, feet hip-width apart, hands on hips, fingers splayed and knees slightly bent and relaxed.

Next

With tummy tucked in, smoothly rotate your hips in a circle – to the left, to the back, to the right and then return to the centre. Repeat 8–10 times then switch direction. Repeat another 8–10 times.

Torso Twist with Bar

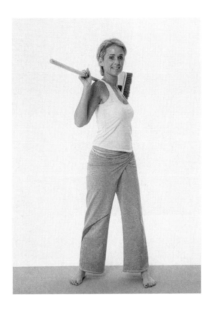

You will need some kind of a pole for this – a broom handle is perfect. This stretch loosens and trains the waist muscles, thus helping to stabilize your upper body. The twist can be hard on your knees, but you won't damage them if you make sure that the entire lower half of your body – from the pelvis to the feet – remains facing forward throughout, with knees relaxed and very slightly bent. Take care to control the twist from your shoulders to your waist. This is the area of your body that is worked during all oblique curls and it is important to make sure it is stretched and under control.

Begin

Stand with your legs hip-width apart, feet facing directly forward, knees relaxed and slightly bent. Place the pole behind your head against the top of your shoulders. Hold it loosely, with your palms facing forward. Pull your abs in and up as if they are connected to the crown of your head and to the ceiling beyond and hold them in that position throughout the stretch – this is your centre.

Next

Slowly twist at the waist so that your upper half turns to the left. Your lower half, from the hips through to the knees and feet, must stay facing forward. Hold. Return to the centre and repeat to the right. Do 8–10 stretches on both sides.

Stand Up and Stretch

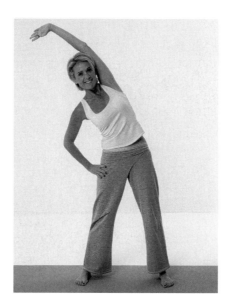

This stretch warms up the muscles at the side of the waist.

Begin

Stand upright, your back stretched and tall, your legs hip-width apart. Bend your knees just a little, put your right hand on your right thigh and reach up with left arm. Keep head, neck and shoulders aligned in a natural position. Do not raise the chin – keep it tucked in a little.

Next

Slowly stretch over to your right side, your left arm still held up. You'll feel your waist stretching. Hold then relax.

Repeat on the other side. Do 8–10 stretches on both sides, holding the stretch for a count of 8–10 between sets of reps.

Floor Twist and Stretch

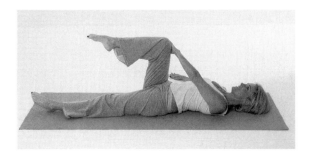

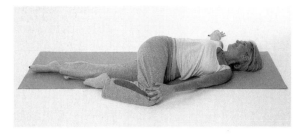

This exercise stretches the muscles of your hips and lower back.

Begin

Lie full length and relaxed on the floor, your arms loosely stretched down the sides of your body. Lift your right knee up partly towards your chest so the thigh is more or less vertical and your lower leg horizontal with the floor. Place your left hand on the outside of your right thigh just above the knee.

Next

Keeping both shoulders and upper back down against the floor as much as possible, use your left hand to bring your right knee across your body towards the opposite side. You will feel your hip muscle stretching. Now push that knee even further down towards the floor, allowing your right shoulder to move up off the floor only as much as necessary. Feel that long stretch expanding into your lower back. Hold then relax. Repeat on the other side.

Curl Up and Stretch

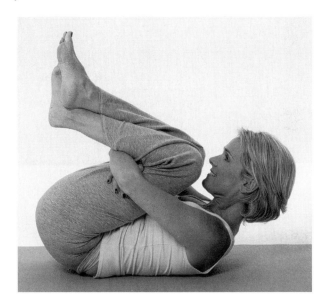

This exercise stretches your entire back and is therefore ideal to finish on.

Begin

Lie on your back, knees raised, feet flat on the ground. Clasp your hands together behind your knees and bring your knees up towards your chest.

Next

Now imagine that you are a hedgehog. Exhale while smoothly coming up as if into a curl, bringing your head and shoulders close to your knees. Your back should feel stretched. Hold then relax.

Nicki Waterman's Flat Stomach Plan

CHAPTER TWO

Stage 1: Beginner's Curls

The basics

You've warmed up – now you're ready to do your first curl. However, before you begin, there are a few basics you need to familiarize yourself with. Begin by getting into the correct basic position (shown on page 14), then go on to study the Top Tips for Doing the Curl (page 15) and How to Breathe (page 16).

At Rest Position

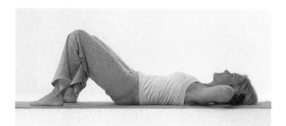

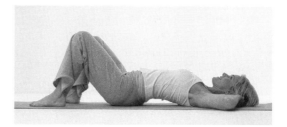

Some people call this position neutral. It is the position in which your body is aligned correctly to do curls and the basic position that should be maintained throughout the exercises (unless instructed otherwise).

1. Lie on your back with your knees bent, feet flat on the floor and hip-width apart. Your knees must be a reasonable distance from your buttocks, so you feel comfortable and relaxed.
2. Keep your shoulders relaxed and down and, with elbows at right angles to your head, rest your head in your unclasped hands.
3. Press your pelvis into the floor as far as possible.
4. Now push up gently, feeling your pelvis tilt away from the floor so that there's a gap between the floor and your lower back. If you could see yourself in profile, you would be able to see this gap. (It's sufficient to allow someone to slide their hands and arms right through to the other side.) This is the arched position or low-back curve.
5. Gently rock back and forth between the flat back and the arched position until you can feel your body settling some where between the two. Your pelvis should now be in a comfortable, balanced position. It is important to practise this and adjust the position of your body until you get it right.

Nicki Waterman's Flat Stomach Plan

Top tips for doing the curl

These guidelines will help you get the most out of your ab routine.

1. Move in a smooth, controlled manner. If you find yourself jerking or getting into the wrong position, stop, focus and start again.
2. Let your abs do the work, not your neck. The curl must come from your stomach region. A common mistake is to interlock fingers or clasp hands behind your neck and haul your head up. Instead, support your head by using your hands as a cradle.
3. During curls where the head is not supported, tuck your chin in a little, allowing the neck muscles to do their work.
4. Avoid the S-bend. Keep head, neck and shoulders aligned in a natural position. Don't look up at the ceiling.
5. To protect your spine and stabilize your pelvis, imagine that you're lengthening your back towards the floor when lifting.
6. Try not to rise more than 30–45 degrees from the floor. More, and you'll be working your hip flexor muscles.
7. Exhale as you lift. Try to pull your tummy in towards your spine and up into your ribs.
8. Use a hand to check the position of your abs – don't allow your tummy to stick out.
9. When doing curls with twists or rotations, first lean forward a little to bring the ribcage towards your pelvis. Then lead with your shoulder and keep the elbows back.

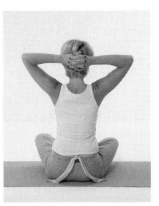

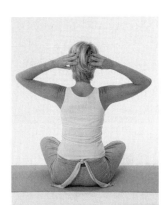

How to Breathe

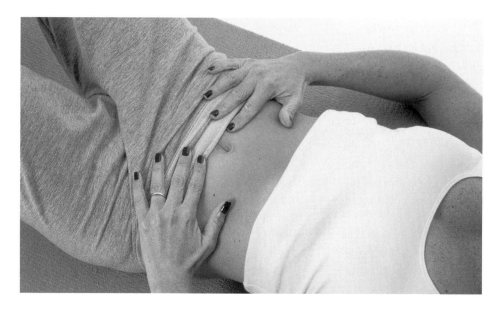

Everyone can breathe, can't they? Actually no! At least, not well enough to gain the optimum from exercise. Learning to breathe correctly during tummy exercises has to be learned and practised. It's important to get it right before you begin because correct breathing has a direct effect on whether you can hold your tummy in and up during the lifting stage of the curl.

You will notice that when we inhale – try it now – the tummy naturally tends to stick out and as we exhale it goes back in. For curls, where the aim is to flatten the tummy and strengthen the abs, we must be able to use and control this breathing pattern to our advantage.

The key to curling is to breathe out during each lift and pull the tummy further in and up

1. Lie on the floor in the basic At Rest position. Instead of having your hands under your head, spread your fingers across your tummy with your thumbs approximately at the bottom of your ribcage (diaphragm) and your middle fingers pointing towards, but not touching, your belly button. Your shoulders should be down on the floor and relaxed. Take a deep breath in.
2. Now breathe out. As you exhale, note the direction your tummy moves. It should flatten slightly.
3. Breathe in. Notice that your belly goes out, or sticks up.
4. Continue breathing in and out, but now exaggerate the pattern so that you can tell the difference. As you exhale, concentrate. Use your abdominal muscles to press your stomach down even further. As you inhale, make your stomach stick out more.

   Continue practising this until you are very aware of how your breathing works in relation to your tummy. The purpose of curling is to utilize the movement of your abs during *exhalation*.

Now that you feel comfortable with your body's posture and position while doing curls, practise the first curl using this breathing technique.

Ab Breathing

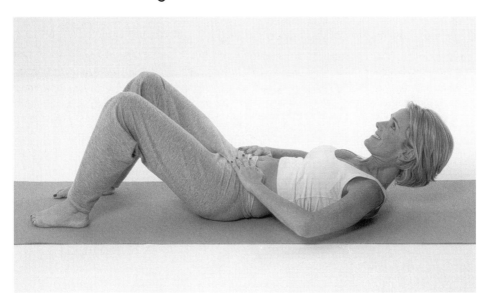

Begin

With elbows resting on the ground at about mid-chest position, place your splayed fingers across your tummy. You will probably feel the top of your pelvic girdle with the heel of your hands and your thumbs will be level with the bottom of your diaphragm. Take a deep breath and feel your abs tightening as you prepare to lift.

Next

Exhale, while pulling your tummy muscles in and upwards. At the same time, slowly curl your spine forward, lifting your shoulders and ribcage. You will feel your mid and lower back lengthening towards the floor, to stabilize your pelvis and protect your spine. Remember to keep your head, neck and shoulders in their basic natural alignment – don't jerk your head forward. Continue to lift while your stomach remains flat – you will feel this with your fingers. As soon as your stomach starts to curl, stop. Return to the At Rest position and repeat.

Continue doing as many repetitions as you can manage, until you are perfectly comfortable with it. You will notice that it is the simultaneous exhalation and pulling in and up of the tummy muscles that naturally starts the curl.

Tip:

Don't move on to the Stage 2 exercises until the ab-breathing technique becomes second nature to you. You'll find that after a while you will automatically breathe out and pull your tummy in and up at the start of each lift. Once you reach this point, you won't need to concentrate. Correct breathing will be automatic as you move nicely into the basic curl.

Do you want fab abs?

If so, try my trademark string waistband. I make all my clients wear a piece of string around their waist when exercising. It is tied when the tummy muscles are tight. If the muscles then slack off, the tightening string reminds the wearer to pull them back in again.

The Stage 1 Routine

Now you are ready to move on to your first curl – the Ab Curl. At first, do the minimum number of repetitions suggested. If you feel tired, or that you can't continue, try just a couple more before stopping. It doesn't hurt to push yourself just a little and it won't be long before you start to get stronger and are able to do the maximum number of reps suggested for each exercise. Ideally, you want to be able to complete at least two successive sets of 8–16 reps nice and smoothly, without resting.

IMPORTANT

You might feel a little stiffness or tiredness to start with, but you shouldn't feel pain or real discomfort during any particular curl. If you do, stop at once. Try again later with some easier exercises to build up your strength before getting back to the one where you felt discomfort. If the pain persists, see your doctor.

Ab Curl

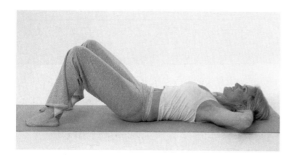

Tip:

If you feel your stomach protruding during the curl, stop. Make a conscious effort to pull it in and up and then continue with the exercise. The purpose of a curl is to train your stomach to be flat.

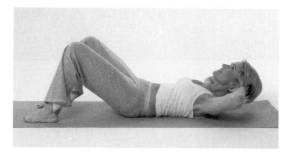

Begin

Get into the At Rest, or basic, position. Lie flat on your back on the floor. Raise your knees, place your feet flat on the floor, hip-width apart and at a comfortable distance from your buttocks. Ensure your pelvis is in the correct position and is neither too flat nor too raised (see page 14). With elbows on the floor at right angles to your head, cradle your head in your hands – i.e. avoid clasping or interlocking your fingers behind your neck. Inhale deeply and prepare to lift.

Next

Remembering to use the basic ab breathing technique, exhale, pulling your tummy in and up. This will start to smoothly lift your shoulders and ribcage off the floor. Keep your shoulders back and relaxed, head cradled in hands, elbows and arms still level and at right angles to your head. Don't strain or try to sit up. Go as far up as is comfortable while keeping your tummy flat and your lower spine pressed against the floor. Your feet should not move.

Return to the basic position and repeat. 4–8 reps will be enough to start with. Gradually work up to two sets of 8–16 reps.

Nicki Waterman's Flat Stomach Plan

Oblique Curl

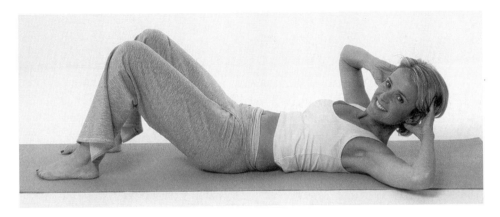

Tips:

Lift before adding the twist. Exhale on the lift, pulling your tummy in and up. Lead with the shoulder and ribcage, not the elbow or you won't work the oblique muscles. Make sure your tummy – particularly the lower part – is not protruding.

The obliques are the muscles that give us that much admired slim and narrow waist. They stretch from the outside of the ribcage diagonally to the pelvis.

Begin

Lie flat on your back in the basic position, head resting in hands, pelvis level, knees raised and feet flat at a comfortable distance from the buttocks. Cradle your head in your hands. Now imagine that your tummy is sinking into your back and keep that feeling in your mind as you proceed.

Next

Come up into the Ab Curl and, as you do, add a twist by bringing one shoulder and the ribcage towards – though not reaching – the opposite knee. Make sure that you keep your elbow relaxed and in line with the shoulder, so that the twist comes from the waist. Remember, it is your obliques that you are working, so visualize the move and think oblique.

Return to the basic position and repeat with the other shoulder. Start with 4–8 reps to each side and work up gradually to two sets of 8–16 reps.

Ab Stretch

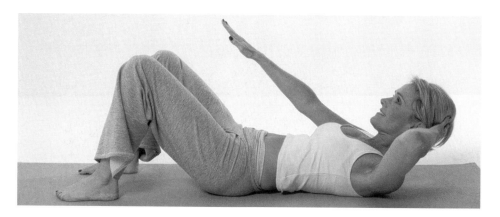

Tips:

As you lift, the elbow and upper arm that are supporting your head will leave the floor but make sure you don't use your elbow to lever your head up. Don't pull your pelvis into a flat back position as you lift. You should feel your abs compressing and your back lengthening towards the floor.

Just one hand supports your head while you follow the other hand into this stretch.

Begin

With elbow and upper arm at right angles to your head, rest your head in one hand. Raise the other arm level and parallel to one knee, hand stretched out as if aiming beyond. Make sure your pelvis is in the basic position.

Next

Exhale while you use the abs to lift yourself into the curl, reaching your raised arm past your knees. Keep your arm straight and your head in the basic position. Let your eyes focus over the top of your raised hand so that your top half – from your waist to the top of your head – lifts nice and smoothly as one. Your elbow and upper arm will leave the ground.

Return to the beginning and repeat. Start with 4 reps, building up to two sets of 8–16 reps. Repeat with the other arm. Do an equal number of reps on both sides.

Stretch and Curl

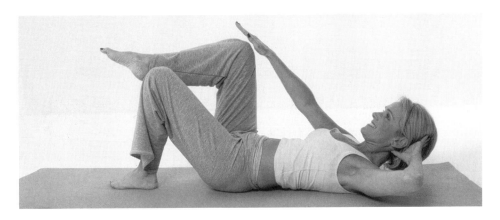

Tips:
With your head supported on only one hand there might be a tendency for your head to jerk up, so concentrate on holding it in the basic position. The aim of this exercise is to focus on holding your stomach as flat as possible throughout, so concentrate on that.

Begin
As in the previous exercise, start with your elbow and upper arm at right angles to your head and rest your head in just one hand. Raise the other arm level and parallel to one knee, hand stretched out as if aiming beyond. Make sure your pelvis is in the basic position. Breathe in deeply, focusing on exhaling and pulling in your abs. Do this three or four times. At the same time, to reinforce that flat stomach feeling, work on letting your torso sink towards your back and up into ribcage.

Next
As in the previous exercise, exhale while you use the abs to lift yourself into the curl, reaching your raised arm past your knees. Keep your arm straight and your head in the basic position. Let your eyes focus over the top of your raised hand so that your top half – from your waist to the top of your head – lifts nice and smoothly as one. Your elbow and upper arm will leave the ground. Now here's the difference – as you lift, bring the knee you are aiming over with your hand in towards your chest. Try to imagine that your pubic bone is also coming towards your chest along with the knee.

Return to the starting position and repeat. Do 4 reps, working up to two sets of 8. Repeat with the opposite arm and knee, doing the same number of reps.

Unsupported Curl

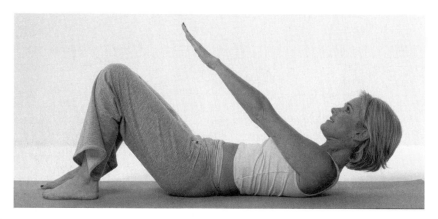

Tips:

Initially, unsupported curls are not easy. Don't worry if you can't manage more than a couple to start with. With practice, your neck muscles will strengthen and you'll be able to do two sets of 8 reps in due course. If you find it impossible to do it without your head jerking all over the place, try using your hands as usual until you are up in the curl, then release them and hold away for a moment, replacing them behind your head as you uncurl back down again.

Now that you are familiar with where your head should be throughout a curl, you are ready to do your first unsupported one. This means letting your neck muscles support the weight of your head instead of your hands. To help, bring your chin down slightly. (Don't take it too far though or you will feel a strain at the back of your neck.)

Begin

Start in the basic position, knees up and feet flat on floor, hip-width apart and at a comfortable distance from your buttocks. Now, instead of cradling your head in your hands, lay your arms down by your sides, palms down. Get your breathing right, taking a deep breath as you prepare to lift your shoulders.

Next

Exhale as you move into the lift, letting your chin drop slightly down to support the weight of your head while smoothly moving your arms forward in a straight line, aiming above your knees. Keep that tummy tucked in nice and flat throughout as you feel your back curl away from the floor.

Return to the starting position and repeat. Do 4 reps, working up to two sets of 8.

Cross and Curl

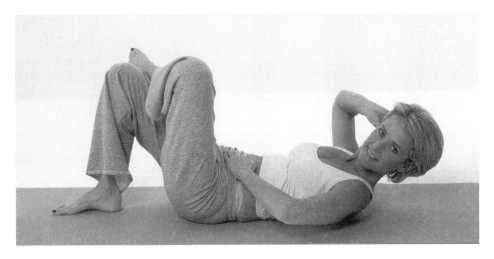

Tip:

Feel the rotation start at the waist so that the whole of the upper torso moves as one fluid unit. It's important to keep the elbow of the arm supporting the head back and relaxed.

Begin

Start in the basic position with knees raised, feet flat on the ground hip-width apart and at a comfortable distance from your buttocks. Bring one leg up and place the ankle on the opposite thigh just above the knee. Rest your head in the opposite hand to the raised leg and lay your other hand flat on your tummy, fingers spread. Let both elbows rest on the ground to start. Breathe in deeply.

Next

Let your breath out smoothly as you come up into the curl and, as you do so, start to twist by lifting and rotating the shoulder of the arm supporting the head, and your ribcage, towards the raised knee. Don't swing your elbow forward or you will find that you are pulling on your neck.

Return to the starting position and repeat. Do 4–8 reps, working up to two sets of 8–16. Repeat, using the other knee and arm, making sure that you do an equal number of reps on both sides.

After each curl workout go to page 75 for your cool-down exercises

CHAPTER THREE

Stage 2:
Intermediate Curls

Don't start with these more advanced curls until you are really comfortable with all the exercises in Stage 1. Once you've mastered the Stage 1 exercises you will be stronger and ready to try something tougher. Once you're ready to move on to Stage 2, take it slowly and start with the minimum number of reps suggested, allowing your body to adapt. If you take your time, you won't feel sore. If anything hurts – stop and try again later. If you still feel pain, see your doctor.

Make sure you review the correct breathing technique before moving on – although if you're really familiar with Stage 1 and are getting it right, it should be second nature to you. If in doubt, try the How to Breathe exercise again (see page 16).

Tip:
As you do these curls, visualize what your body is doing. Focus on your abs and how they feel – visualize your tummy flattening as the muscles work.

Remember, no matter how advanced you feel you are, always do a warm up first (see page 1)

Reverse Curl

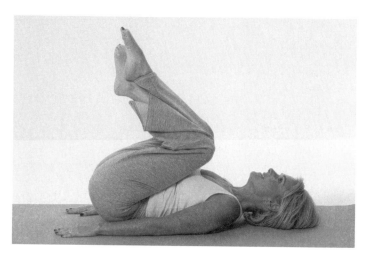

Tip:
Keep your actions smooth – don't jerk the knees back and forth or rock on your tailbone.

In this curl, the usual action of lifting the upper body is reversed and instead the pelvis is brought towards the ribcage.

Begin

Lie flat, with knees up and bent as close to your chest as possible, calves resting on your thighs, ankles crossed. Let your legs feel relaxed and heavy.

Your arms should be lying on the floor along your sides, palms facing down so you can push *gently* if necessary (but no – you don't heave yourself up on your arms).

Next

Breathe in deeply. Now exhale, at the same time pressing your tummy in and up towards your ribcage while starting to gradually curl up the lower part of your spine. You should feel your pelvis move up towards your ribcage.

Concentrate on curling the spine. It's important that you use the tummy muscles to pull your knees forward and not your leg muscles. If you're doing this correctly, your knees will automatically move closer to your upper body and you'll feel your abs working.

Return to the starting position by smoothly uncurling your spine, letting your tailbone down towards the floor. Repeat. Start with 4–8 reps, working up to 8–16.

Nicki Waterman's Flat Stomach Plan

Leg Lift and Curl

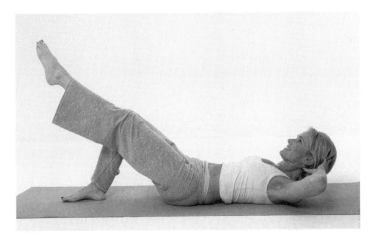

Tip:
During the curl, keep your back lengthened towards the floor and your tummy pulled in. However, don't let your pelvis be pulled into a flat back position.

Begin

Lie down in the basic position, head resting in hands. Now, with knees remaining side by side, raise one leg and extend it fully, without pointing your foot. Breathe in deeply.

Next

Start the curl, simultaneously breathing out and, as you do so, pull the tummy in and up while trying to extend the raised leg, really stretching it. You will feel the rectus abdominus (the long muscle that forms the middle section of your abs between ribcage and pelvis) pulling away from the extended leg towards your ribcage. Keep your elbows back and relaxed. (Obviously as you lift up, your elbows will leave the floor, but don't swing them forward in an effort to make the curl easier or you will drag on your neck.)

Return to the starting position. Do 4–8 reps, working up to two sets of 8–16. Repeat with the other leg raised. Make sure you do the same number of reps on each side.

Leg Lift and Twist

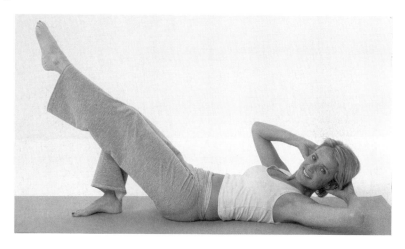

Tip:
Keep both hips and buttocks firmly on the floor – don't move into a roll.

This is similar to the previous exercise but has an added twist.

Begin

Start with your head cradled in your hands, knees together, right leg bent with foot flat on the floor, the left leg stretched.

Next

Using your abs to pull your right shoulder up, twist it towards the extended left leg. Your right elbow will rise, while the left one should remain on the floor. Keep the motion fluid, using a little forward flexion to bring your ribcage towards your pelvis, but make sure that you don't use the raised arm to drag your shoulder forward.

Return to the starting position and repeat. Do 4–8 reps, working up to 8–16. Repeat with the other leg extended. Ensure you do the same number of reps on each side.

Cross Arms and Curl

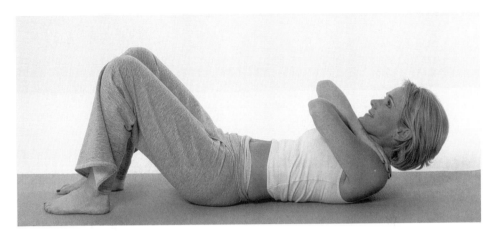

Tip:
Your chin should remain in the same position on your arms. If you feel any neck strain, you're not allowing your abs to do the work.

Begin

Start in the basic position but instead of cradling your head, raise and cross your arms over your chest in the collarbone area, elbows up and each hand on the top of the opposite shoulder. Your chin should rest on your arms where they cross.

Make sure that your pelvis is in the correct basic position and inhale deeply. With your back long and pressed to the floor, you should feel your tummy sink into your back.

Next

Start to lift, exhaling smoothly. Your raised elbows should move towards your thighs while your chin remains resting on your crossed arms. However, don't force your shoulders forward – your abs should be doing the work.

This curl is tough on your neck muscles, so don't try to do too many to start with. Do 4 reps at first, gradually increasing to two sets of 8–16.

Roll Up and Curl

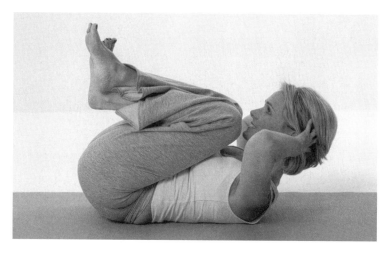

Tip:
Keep the roll up slow and controlled. Don't rock – you're not a ball.

This neat little curl combines the Ab Curl and the Reverse Curl.

Begin

Lie in the basic position, head resting on hands. Bring your knees right up towards your chest and cross your ankles, calves resting on thighs. Your legs should be relaxed and heavy. Feel your tummy muscles pressing down towards your back. Breathe in deeply.

Next

Exhale and lift, curling your spine to bring your ribcage and your knees close together. Try to make a ball of your body but avoid using momentum – the entire curl must come from your abs tightening and flattening. Your face should end up between your knees.

Lower your upper body and repeat. Start with 4–8 reps, working up to two sets of 8–16.

Cross Over and Reach

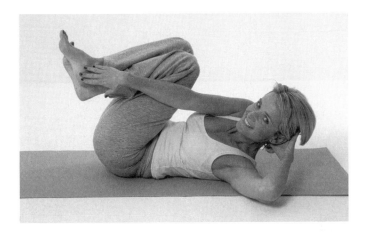

Tip:
Don't do this exercise in a sloppy manner or you won't achieve much. Keep it all fluid. Don't jerk one shoulder forward and the knee in the opposite direction. You should really feel your abs compress and tighten.

This is quite a complicated curl, so don't rush it. Do it one step at a time, thinking about each stage. Eventually, you will be able to do it automatically.

Begin

Start in the same position as the Roll Up and Curl, with head resting in hands, knees up as close to the chest as possible and ankles crossed.

Next

Exhale, move into a curl and, as you do so, bring your right arm forward and across your chest, past the outside of the left knee. Simultaneously, allow the left hip that the right arm is aiming at to twist up towards the armpit of the left arm (which should still be supporting your head). Your feet will slide closer to the raised hand and your knees will move away towards the raised shoulder.

Return to the starting position and repeat. Start with 4 reps, working up to two sets of 8. Repeat on the other side with the same number of reps.

Hands to Knees

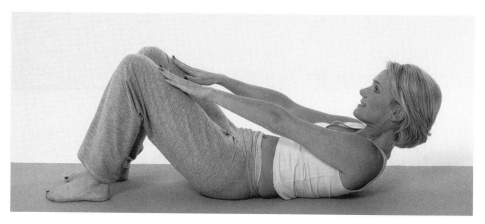

Tips:
Try holding your legs at the top of the curl, using your arms to maintain position while you focus on your stomach, feeling the muscles flatten. As you lift, look over the top of your knees.

This curl is tough on the neck, so take it slowly.

Begin
Lying in the basic position, stretch out your arms and rest your open hands on the front of your thighs. To help support your head, bring your chin down slightly, keeping the neck in line with the spine as much as possible.

Next
Using your abs to lift into a curl, allow your hands to slide up your thighs towards your knees. Try to lift your ribcage as much as possible while keeping your stomach flat and lengthening your back against the floor.

If you feel your tummy muscles sticking up, start again. This time, keep the curl lower. Eventually your abs will get stronger and you will be able to rise higher.

Return to the starting position and repeat. Start with 4–8 reps, working up to two sets of 8–16.

Frog Curl

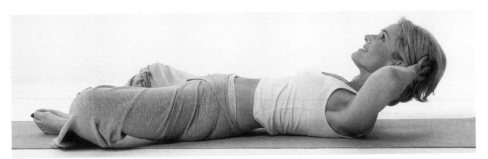

Tips:

You might find this open leg position difficult at first if you don't have enough flexibility in your inner thighs. Try relaxing the upper body after each rep but keep your legs splayed. This will gradually stretch your inner thigh muscles.

With your knees out of normal alignment, your back might rise and curve off the floor. If this happens, focus on lengthening your back and pressing it down while at the same time pulling your abs in and up towards the ribcage.

The position adopted for this curl resembles a swimming frog.

Begin

Lie in the basic position with head resting in hands, but instead of having the knees up, allow them to fall open to the sides with your heels together and your ankles in line with your lower legs. Inhale. Press your tummy in towards your back.

Next

Keeping your pelvis in its correct position, exhale while lifting into a curl. Feel your abs tighten from the pubic area to the ribcage.

Return to the starting position and do 4–8 reps, working up to two sets of 8–16.

Heel Lift and Reach

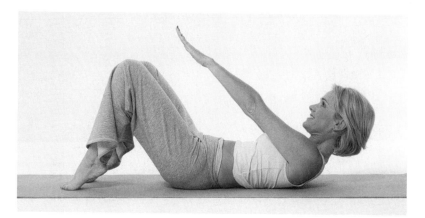

Tips:

This can be hard on your calves – if you get cramp, lower your heels back to the floor and stretch your toes towards the ceiling (keeping heels down). You could practise the heel lift without the curl to strengthen your calf muscles.

This starts off like a standard curl but by lifting the heels it also uses the calf muscles.

Begin

Lie in the basic position with your knees raised and head resting in hands. Focus on lengthening and flattening your back towards the floor and pulling the abs in and up. Take a deep breath.

Next

Exhale as you come into a curl. At the same time, smoothly lift your hands away from your head and reach your arms towards your knees, parallel to the tops of your thighs, simultaneously lifting your heels as high as possible, keeping your toes pressed against the floor. However, don't put your weight on your toes – your weight should be on your hips. You will instantly feel your calves contract.

Return to the starting position and do 4 reps, building up to two sets of 8–16.

Nicki Waterman's Flat Stomach Plan

Twist and Turn

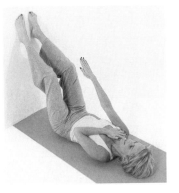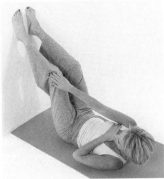

Tips:

Keep your neck in the basic position by moving the head and upper torso as one and looking in the direction of your twist.

Ensure that the twist comes from the shoulder and that side of the ribcage by pointing the shoulder towards the opposite knee. At the same time, keep the abs pulled in to do the lift.

You will need to use a wall for this exercise.

Begin

Start in the basic curl position with your buttocks at a comfortable distance from a wall so that you can put your feet flat up against the wall with your knees slightly bent. Your heels should be higher than your knees. Stretch out your right arm, aiming for the top of your knees. Cross your left hand over your chest, elbow slightly up, and put it on the right shoulder. Inhale.

Next

Exhale, lift smoothly into a curl then twist at the waist, reaching with the stretched right arm for the outside of the left knee. Lay the flat of your right hand against the outside of the left knee. If your pelvis gets out of its correct position, re-rock it until it's right (see At Rest position page 14) and start over.

Return to the starting position and do 8 reps, building up to two sets of 8–16. Reverse arms and repeat on opposite side with an equal number of reps.

Note: After each curl workout go to page 75 for your cool-down exercises

CHAPTER FOUR

Stage 3: Difficult Curls

By now, you know what you're doing where curls are concerned. You automatically breathe correctly, and your pelvis, neck and head stay in their correct basic position during the exercises. You're a lot stronger than when you started your ab programme and your tummy is a lot flatter. Your task now is to maintain the ground you've won through your sheer hard work and to get even fitter and flatter.

Focus now on always being aware of your stomach and keeping your ab muscles tight and firm throughout the day, regardless of what you're doing. Diet will also play a part – don't eat huge meals that will stretch your stomach and bloat you out.

A great benefit of strong abs is that your back will be better supported. If more people had strong stomach muscles, chronic back pain would be less prevalent. However, don't try to run before you can walk. Some of the exercises in this section are pretty hard. If the instructions tell you to start with 4 reps and gradually work up, follow this advice. Make sure you are comfortable at the start of every exercise – if you feel any discomfort, stop, readjust your position and start over. If you find you are unable to get it right, you are probably tired. Stop, take a rest, perhaps for an hour or two, or perhaps wait until the next day. If any back pain is sharp or persists, see your doctor.

You'll know you have mastered Stage 3 when you can do all the reps suggested easily and without resting. You might wish to stay at this stage for a while by doing more reps than suggested before moving on to Stage 4.

Meanwhile, here you are, having mastered Stages 1 and 2 and ready to graduate to Stage 3 – so you should feel proud of yourself, not to mention a great deal stronger and fitter.

Remember, only go as fast as you feel is right for you. You've already achieved a lot through your dedicated hard work – but you can achieve a lot more.

Always warm up and stretch first before any workout session

Nicki Waterman's Flat Stomach Plan

Backward Curl

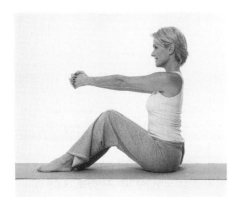 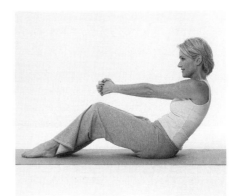

Tips:

Don't rock on your bottom. Use your rounded back to keep you balanced as you move back, not the muscles at the top of your thighs (the hip flexors). Keep your tummy muscles lifted and your stomach tucked in.

Begin

Sit on the floor with your knees raised, your feet hip-width apart and at a comfortable distance from your buttocks, and imagine you are sitting upright in a straight-backed chair. Now stretch your arms out, parallel with the floor, hands clasped loosely. Make your back even straighter and taller. Imagine something is stretching you from your tailbone to the crown of your head. Breathe in deeply and pull your tummy muscles in. Feel your abs vanish deep inside your ribcage.

Next

Making sure that you keep that lift in the middle, exhale while smoothly rounding your spine. The idea is to put more of your buttocks on the floor. You will feel your pelvis moving down into a position where it feels like a pivot – but don't rock on it. Keep on smoothly rounding your spine and you'll feel your upper torso moving back. Don't go too far back or you won't keep that tummy flat.

Return to the starting position and repeat. Do 4–8 reps, working up to two sets of 8–16.

Stretch Up and Reach

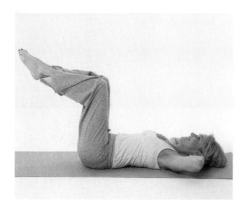 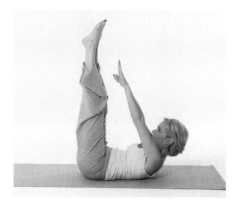

Tips:

Looking along your arms to the tips of your fingers as you lift will help keep your head in the correct position. Lower your knees towards your torso when returning to the starting position.

Begin

Lie on the floor in the basic position, head cradled in hands. Now raise your legs so that your knees are bent and over your hips and your lower legs are slightly elevated. This should be comfortable – if you feel any strain in your back, try bending the knees slightly more. Keep your hips and lower back on the floor throughout. Inhale deeply.

Next

Exhale as you lift, stretching both arms towards your feet. At the same time, straighten your knees and push the feet up towards the ceiling, keeping them flat, not pointed. The effort in the lift must come from the long tummy muscles, bringing the ribcage and pubic area closer together.

Return to the starting position and repeat. Do 4–8 reps, gradually increasing to two sets of 8–16.

Lift, Curl and Cross

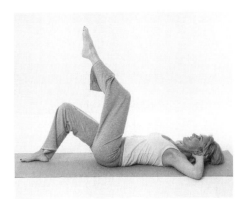 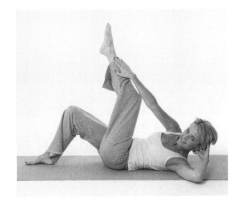

Tips:
Concentrate on what your abs are doing throughout the move. Keep the raised leg in the same position above the hips – don't allow it to fall towards the chest. The knee should be nicely relaxed.

Begin

Lie on your back in the basic position, knees bent and feet flat on the floor, hip-width apart. Cradle your head in your hands and lift it slightly, keeping elbows on the floor at right angles to your head.

Raise your left leg, keeping your knee bent. Don't change the position of the right leg and foot.

Next

Now do an Ab Curl and, leading from the shoulder, add a twist from the waist. Your head will lift and turn. As you twist, extend the right arm towards the outside of the raised left foot. Stretch that arm out as far as you can – but take care not to use your raised shoulder or the supporting left arm on the floor to pull you through. All the effort must be done by your abs as you pull them in nice and tight. Your arm, shoulder and ribcage should move smoothly as one.

Return to the starting position and repeat. Do 8 reps, gradually working up to two sets of 8–16. Repeat on other side, making sure you do the same number of reps.

Head and Toe

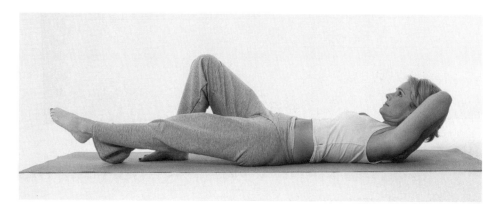

Tip:

It is very easy to pull your elbows forward and use the arms to help you lift – but don't be tempted. If you keep your elbows relaxed and back, you can focus on the correct source of strength for this exercise – your abs.

Begin

Lie flat on your back in the basic position. Now move your hands so that the palms are flat against the top of your back, pointing downwards towards your shoulder blades, and your head is resting on your lower arms. (The top of your head should be about level with your elbows.)

Keeping your thighs together and parallel, extend your right leg straight out, so it is a few inches off the floor. Inhale deeply.

Next

Exhale, pulling your abs up and back. Lift your shoulders in a curl (using your abs) and, at the same time, stretch your extended leg even further forward. Keep it stretched while maintaining the tension in the abs. Make sure that your pelvis remains in the basic position.

Return to the starting position and repeat. Do 4–8 reps, working up to two sets of 8–16 reps. Repeat with the other leg, doing the same number of reps on each side.

Head-Supported Twist

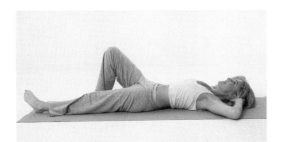

Tip:

It's not easy to hold the extended leg low and straight. It will help if you focus on stretching the leg rather than lifting it.

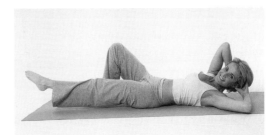

This exercise works the side abdominals (waist).

Begin

Start in the basic position. Now move your right hand to lie flat in the centre of your back, fingers towards the shoulder blade (as in the previous curl, Head and Toe). The fingers of the left hand cradle the head in its normal position, left elbow at right angles and resting on the floor. Now extend your left leg fully in a straight line, parallel to the right leg (which remains with knee bent up, foot flat on floor).

Next

Start with a basic Ab Curl, but add a twist by bringing the right shoulder towards the extended left leg. Simultaneously, lift the extended leg just a few inches off the floor, keeping it level and stretched out. The bottom of your extended calf should be about level with the top of your sneakers.

Return to the starting position and repeat. Do 8 reps, working up to two sets of 8–16. Repeat on the other side, doing an equal number of reps on each side.

Reach Out and Curl

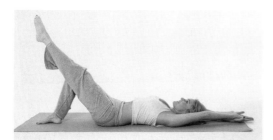

Tip:
This looks easy but is quite difficult, so start with a small number of reps until you can comfortably do more.

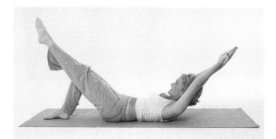

This exercise is a tough one and really works those abs.

Begin

Lie in the basic position but with your arms extended above your head, hands crossed at wrist, upper arms close to ears. (Your head will be supported by the upper arms during the lift.) Keep your shoulders relaxed and comfortable. Ensure your pelvis is in the right position. Raise your left leg, keeping thighs parallel, knees touching. Inhale deeply.

Next

Exhale as you smoothly lift your upper body and stretch that left leg. It won't actually move, but mentally imagine it stretching. The idea is to keep the body long and your tummy flat throughout.

Return to the starting position and repeat. Do 4 reps, gradually working up to two sets of 8–12. Repeat with the other leg. Do the same number of reps on each side.

Wall Curl

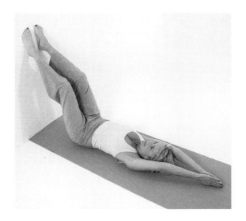 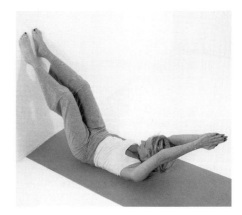

Tip:

This is a hard curl, so take it slowly with reps at first, only doing more as you get stronger.

In this exercise you use a wall to support your legs and help keep your pelvis in its basic position.

Begin

Lie on your back at a distance from the wall that allows you to put your feet up against it at an angle slightly higher than your knees. You should feel comfortable and relaxed. Stretch your arms straight behind your head alongside your ears, wrists touching on palm side and fingers extended. Your head will be supported by the inner part of your upper arms. Take a deep breath and start to flatten the stomach.

Next

Exhale while lifting your head and upper torso smoothly. You will feel your abs really working hard. Make sure that your shoulders stay back in line with your head and neck by keeping your arms next to your ears.

Return to the starting position and repeat. Do 4 reps, working up to two sets of 8–16 reps.

Hug Curl

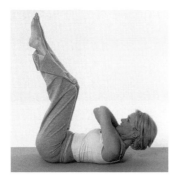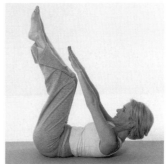

Tips:

This is a tough curl to hold so make sure you go through each stage carefully. When you are balanced with hands and legs up, press your abs hard down to the floor – imagine your navel is nailed to the mat – to keep yourself in place. Don't roll back down until your hands are fully in place again on your shoulders. Keep your neck in line, don't jerk your head forward. Throughout, be aware that your abs are doing all the work, so focus on that action.

Begin

Lie on your back and get your pelvis into the correct basic position. Cross your arms over your chest, putting each hand flat on the opposite shoulder, elbows raised. Lift your legs up, knees bent above tummy and with lower legs at a slope towards ceiling. Inhale and exhale deeply, pulling the tummy muscles in and up as you go into a smooth lift, aiming your elbows at your knees. This is the starting position. Hold it briefly.

Next

Extend your arms out past your knees, seeing how far you can stretch them while at the same time keeping your abs in and flat. Your legs should stay in the same position. You're not rolling into a ball, but pulling up with your abdominal muscles.

Still holding this position, bring your arms slowly back down to cross over on your chest, hands on opposite shoulders. Now roll yourself back to the floor. Take a rest, legs still up, before doing another.

Repeat, starting with 4 reps. Gradually work up to two sets of 8–12 reps.

Holding Hands

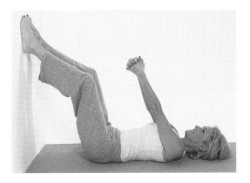

Tip:
Imagining a 'friend' is helping to pull you up really does help. It seems to make the curl easier, allowing you to focus on keeping your tummy muscles nice and flat.

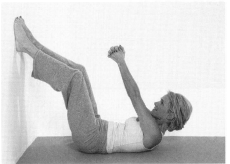

This exercise involves a wall and an imaginary partner who is lending a helping hand.

Begin

Lie down at a comfortable distance from the wall, place your feet on the wall hip-width apart and knees slightly bent, lower legs on a slight upward slope. Get into a position where you feel relaxed and comfortable. Extend your arms towards your knees at an angle parallel to your thighs and clasp your hands.

Next

Come up into the curl and, as you do so, visualize your imaginary friend coming through the wall and pulling you up towards him. Your head isn't supported, so there is a temptation to jerk your head and shoulders forward to help the lift. Resist this and keep everything in line.

Return to the starting position and repeat. Start with 4 reps, working up to two sets of 8–16.

After each curl workout go to page 75 for your cool-down exercises

CHAPTER FIVE

Stage 4:
Tough Curls

If you have made it this far you are entitled to feel very pleased with yourself. You have worked hard and as a result you no doubt have a flat stomach and are fitter, leaner and stronger. In addition, your posture should have improved immeasurably. So much back trouble is due to weak tummy muscles and the added strength at the front means your back is also stronger and better supported.

However, as with all forms of exercise, there is always a further challenge and the following exercises will take you to a new level. Don't attempt them until you feel you are fully ready – and take it easy at first. Start with just a few reps (I suggest 4), working up to two sets of 8–16 reps without resting between sets.

Always warm up and stretch first before any workout session

Fist Curl

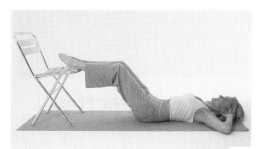

Tip:
Tempting as it is, do not use your feet and shoulders to pull yourself up into the curl – use your abs.

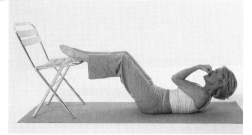

Use a chair for this exercise. Any chair will do, but the most suitable is the kind with a gap at the front between seat and crossbar for you to hook your heels into.

Begin
With your thighs at a 45-degree angle, rest your heels comfortably on the chair, your head cradled in your hands. Make sure your pelvis is in the correct basic position. Breathe in deeply and pull your tummy muscles in and up.

Next
Exhale as you start to lift, at the same time bringing your arms up, elbows bent and hands in loose fists, as if completing a chest or pec press. (This exercise also works the pectoral, or chest, muscles.) Press your elbows towards each other, squeezing your arms together. Keep your shoulders back, your head and neck correctly aligned and your back lifted.

Return to the starting position and repeat. Do 4 reps, gradually working up to two sets of 8–12 reps.

Box and Curl

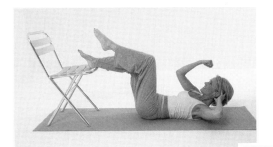

Tip:
This is a tough exercise, so only stay up as long as you are able without straining. Keep your tummy flat throughout and maintain correct breathing.

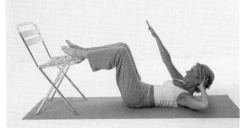

This exercise also requires a chair.

Begin
With your heels up and resting on a chair, cradle your head in your left hand. (The elbow will be further back than usual to support the shoulder and arm swing.) Raise your right arm and bend it slightly, fist loosely clenched. Lift your left heel off the chair so that your left thigh is vertical, knee still bent. Hold. Now bring your right shoulder forward, arm still raised. This is your starting position. It sounds complicated, but the first photograph illustrates it clearly.

Next
As you lift your right shoulder further, extend the right arm towards your raised left leg. However, at the same time, you will be lowering that leg back to the chair, heel back in place next to its partner so your arm will be chasing the leg (but slowly and in a controlled way). Reach across with that arm as far as you can, while maintaining a flat tummy. Make sure your hips and pelvis stay flat on the floor in the correct position.

Return to the starting position – making sure that your abs stay nice and flat – and repeat. Do 4 reps, gradually working up to two sets of 8–12. Return to the floor, rest and then do the same number of reps on the other side.

Side Curl — stage 1

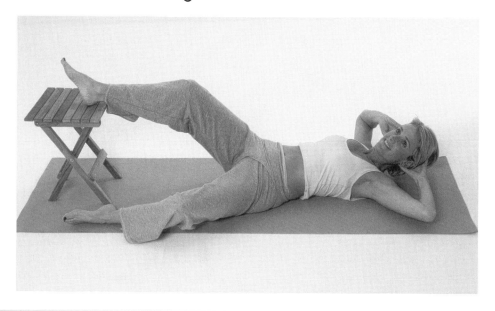

This curl uses a stool (you can use a chair or a sofa, but it must be very low). The exercise is in two parts, each of which must be followed through to make one complete rep – so read it carefully before you start.

1st STAGE:

Begin

Lie on your back in the basic curl position, head cradled loosely in hands, but with elbows slightly further back to support an oblique lift. Rest your right leg on a pouffe with the left leg on the floor, knee loosely bent and at a comfortable angle. Now bring the right side of your torso up so that you are not fully on one side, nor fully on your back but your weight is somewhere between the two. Inhale as you prepare for the curl.

Next

Exhale as you swing your right arm forward – using your abs to make the move rather than your shoulders or the weight of your arm. The idea is to aim your right underarm – not the elbow – towards your right hip.

Return to the starting position and repeat, doing 4 reps.

Side Curl – stage 2

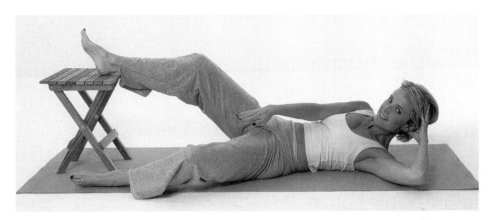

Tip:
Keep your hips and pelvis stable and in the same position throughout for maximum results. Use your abs for the lift and your outstretched arm only as a guide – not as a tool to swing yourself forward.

2nd STAGE:

Begin

With your back pressed against the floor and head resting on your right arm, stretch your left arm out parallel with your right (raised) thigh. Breathe in and tighten your abs.

Next

Exhale and lift, at the same time reaching across your body with your left arm towards your raised right leg. Keep your hips down in the same position.

Return to the floor and repeat, doing 4 reps.

Repeat the entire sequence of two stages on the other side, doing an equal number of reps on both sides. Start with 4 reps for each stage and work up to two sets of 8–16 reps on each side.

Thigh Curls

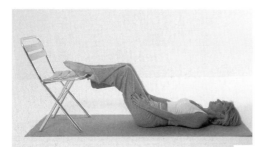

Tip:
Remember, it's your abs that are doing the lifting, not your shoulders, so keep them back. Don't be tempted to do this exercise quickly – it's not a race.

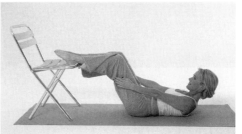

This is another chair exercise, but this time it is a straightforward curl that you count along to.

Begin
Start in the basic curl position but with both heels resting on a chair, legs together, knees bent, thighs at a 45-degree angle. With your upper arms lying alongside your ribs, place your hands on the sides of your thighs. Breathe in.

Next
Exhale, bringing your chin down a little to help support your head. As you start the lift, slide your arms up your thighs, going as high as you can without allowing your back off the floor. Lift up on counts 1 and 2, hold on count 3 and return to the starting position on count 4. Keep the movement nice and smooth as you curl and uncurl – don't jerk.

Repeat, doing 4 reps. Gradually work up to two sets of 8–16.

Lift and Twist

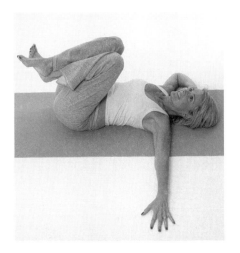 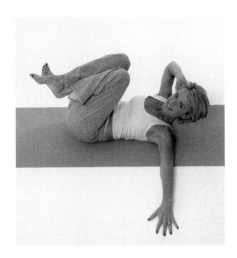

Tip:
Don't roll your torso or swing your legs over. Keep your hips flat on the floor.

Begin

Lie in the basic curl position, but with your right hand lightly supporting your head, the left arm stretched out on the floor at right angles to your body (you will find that this outstretched arm helps stabilize your hips to keep them flat on the floor). Cross your ankles and bend your knees, lifting your legs up and towards your chest as high as possible, without letting your tailbone and lower back leave the floor. Inhale, ensuring that your abs are pulled in and flat.

Next

Exhale, at the same time lifting your right shoulder and ribcage by using your abs. Move your right arm (the bent one supporting your head) towards your outstretched left arm, taking care not to swing right over, or to use your hand to drag your head over. Your hips must stay in place.

Do 4 reps, increasing to two sets of 8–16. Repeat on the other side, doing the same number of reps.

Double Oblique

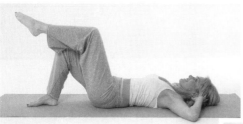

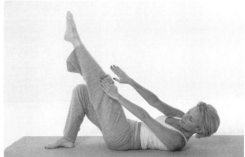

Tip:
It's tempting to jerk your head back and forth with the lift so concentrate on keeping it in its basic position. Remember, the lift and twist come from the abs, not from your shoulders or the forward swing of your arms.

Begin
Lie on the floor in the basic curl position, head lightly cradled in hands with your knees up and feet flat on floor in line with your hips. Now raise your left leg, keeping both knees level but the left foot slightly higher. Bring your chin down slightly to help support your head. Breathe in.

Next
Exhale, contracting your abs down and back into the ribcage as you lift. Simultaneously, twist from the waist, aiming your right shoulder over and towards the raised leg and, in a fluid move-ment, stretch your raised leg and swing your arms forward to reach beyond the outside of the raised leg.

Return to the starting position and repeat. Do 4 reps, gradually working up to two sets of 8–16. Repeat on the other side, doing the same number of reps.

Rope Curl

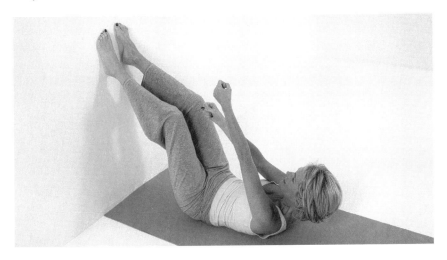

Tip:

Tuck your chin in and don't bring your head forward or allow it to fall back.

You need a wall and a bit of imagination for this curl.

Begin

Lie on the floor in the basic curl position but with your feet flat against a wall, slightly higher than your knees. Your body should feel slightly stretched but not too much so – if you keep your knees at an angle just beyond your buttocks you should get it right. Make sure that your hips are in the correct position.

Now imagine that you are holding a fat rope that dangles down above you. Your loosely clenched fists should be level with your raised knees, grasping that rope. Hold on tight and take a deep breath.

Next

Exhale, pulling your abs in as you prepare to lift. Now pull yourself up the rope to a count of four. Go as far as you can without allowing your lower back to leave the ground. There might be the temptation to press with your feet and buttocks to assist the lift – resist. The lift must come from the contraction of your abs.

Release and unroll smoothly to the floor on a count of four. Repeat, doing 4 reps to start. Work up to two sets of 8–16.

Note: After each curl workout go to page 75 for your cool-down exercises

The best ab move ever

This great curl hits all areas of the tummy region more effectively than any other floor-based exercise. It's a variation of the old bicycling in the air routine (if you remember, in that one, you held your hips up with your hands – not always a good idea) but it's much better. In this exercise, you keep your back parallel with the floor. The idea is to pedal in slow motion, while at the same time twisting your torso and bringing one elbow forward to meet the opposite knee (left elbow to right knee and vice versa). It sounds complicated but with practise you'll soon get it right. In terms of grading, it's up there with a Stage 3 curl so don't attempt it before you're fully prepared and have worked your way through at least Stage 1.

Nicki Waterman's Flat Stomach Plan

The Criss-Cross Bicycle

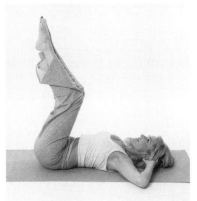 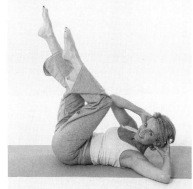

Tips:

Don't rock between your shoulder and hips. The twist should come from the waist, so while part of your back does lift transversely, your knees should stay up and your hips should remain flat on the floor. Remember to exhale on each lift.

Begin

Start in the basic curl position with your lower back pressed into the floor, hands lightly supporting your head, and elbows at right angles to your head. Keeping your hips on the floor, raise your legs and bend your knees towards your chest at a 45-degree angle. Keep your knees above your pelvis, don't let them fall so far forward that you feel any strain in your lower back area.

Next

On an exhalation, lift the upper body off the floor then twist at the waist to bring the right shoulder and elbow towards the left knee, at the same time bringing that knee down to meet it. Then move the left elbow to the right knee, nice and smoothly. Do not lower your shoulders to the floor; keep your torso elevated as you alternate in a slow pedalling motion.

Keep your head supported by both hands, shoulders relaxed. Be conscious of keeping your abs pulled in and back throughout the exercise.

Begin with 4 reps, working up to three sets of 8–12 reps.

Fab Abs Challenge

This section is only for the supremely fit and not to be attempted until you are practised and confident about the strength of your abs and back. Working those tummy muscles is hard and the following exercises prove that it's definitely not a bed of roses for the unfit and less than supple.

Always warm up and stretch first before any workout session

Fab abs routine

Crossed-Wrist Curl

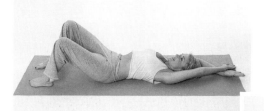

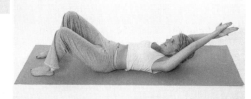

Tip:
Curl as far as you can without straining.
Let your abs do the work.

This is a hard curl so don't overdo it.

Begin

Lie in the basic position, back pressed against the floor, knees raised and feet flat on the floor, hip-width apart. With your upper arms on either side of your head for support, extend your arms above your head (on the floor) and cross your wrists. Your open hands will be overlapping, fingers stretched. Inhale, flattening your abs in and up under the ribcage.

Next

Exhale as you lift, using your abs. Your arms and head will come up smoothly with your shoulders and ribcage in a single unit. Unroll equally smoothly.

Repeat, doing 4 reps. Work up to two sets of 8–16.

Let Go and Reach

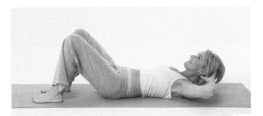

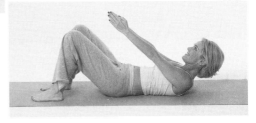

Tips:
Keep your upper body lifted in a curl throughout the exercise. As your arms return to the back of your head prior to going back down, resist the temptation to collapse. It will help if you press your abs down even harder to keep you up in that curl during the final downward move. Don't forget to keep your head in its correct unsupported position.

There are four stages to this curl. It depends on timing and is a really hard one to maintain. Read the instructions carefully and follow each photograph to get the position and the stages right. Practise it slowly first a few times until you can do it smoothly.

Begin
Lie on the floor in the basic position, head lightly resting on fingers, legs hip-width apart and feet flat on the floor at a comfortable distance from your buttocks. Check that your pelvis is in the correct position. Breathe in.

Next
Count 1: Tighten your abs in and up. Exhale. At the same time, come up into a smooth curl. Maintain this.

Count 2: Drop your chin a little towards your chest to help support your head and bring your arms forward parallel with your thighs. Use your abs to reach your arms even further forward beyond your knees, hands outstretched.

Count 3: Maintain your lift as you bring your arms back into their original position with hands behind your head – this requires concentration.

Count 4: Return to the floor and rest – you've earned it.

Do 4 reps to start, gradually working up to two sets of 8–16.

Lying Toe Touches

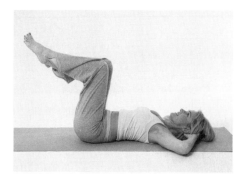 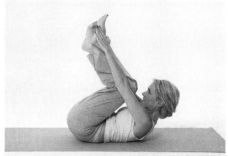

Tips:

If you find this a strain on your back, relax your knees in a bent position over your midriff, but make sure that your buttocks don't go up too far. Keep your eyes above your knees so your head stays in the correct position. To make this even more challenging, use one arm at a time and concentrate on the muscles doing the moving.

This is excellent for giving your upper abs a good workout.

Begin

Lie on your back in the basic position, making sure that the small of your back is pressed to the floor. Your hands will be lightly supporting your head. Raise your legs so that your buttocks are partly lifted, but take care that your tailbone and lower back don't go up. Tighten your abs and take a deep breath.

Next

As you exhale, start to criss-cross your ankles in a scissor movement as you simultaneously curl up and bring your arms forward, stretching them hard towards your toes (drop your chin very slightly to support your head). Pause at the top then slowly lower back to the start.

Do 4 reps and gradually work up to one set of 10–15 reps.

Nicki Waterman's Flat Stomach Plan

One Leg V-Crunches

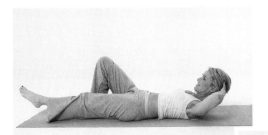

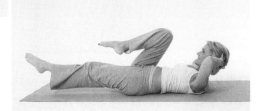

Tip:
Try to keep your shoulders and the outstretched leg up and your abs contracted throughout the entire set of reps. It's tough – but if you've got this far you can do it.

This is a fabulous exercise for working both the upper and lower abs.

Begin

Lie in the basic position, knees bent and feet flat on the floor, your head in your hands and your elbows at right angles. Now straighten your left leg and lift it a few inches off the floor. Hold it there. Tighten your abs hard in and up while you raise up in a partial curl. Hold it and breathe in.

Next

Exhale and, as you do so, bring up the bent knee towards your chest while you rise up to meet it in a curl. Keep your lower back pressed into the floor and use your tummy muscles to continue the upper back lift. Now slowly uncurl back to the start.

Do 4 reps to start, working up to one set of 10–15. Repeat on the other side with your left leg stretched out and raised.

Killer Curl

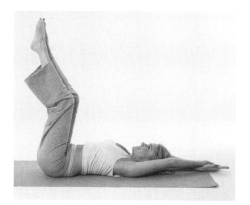 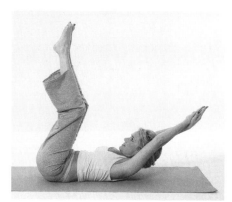

Tip:

Don't allow yourself to 'rock' forwards as you lift, or to rock back down. The movement must be smoothly controlled by the strength in your tummy muscles. If your back feels strained, try this exercise later when your abs are stronger.

Don't attempt this very difficult curl until your abs are in peak condition. It looks easy – but don't be fooled.

Begin

Lie on your back in the basic position but with your arms extended on the floor beyond your head, crossed at the wrist, hands lying loosely on each other. Press your upper arms against your ears and head for support. Now raise your legs, feet in the air and knees slightly bent over your tummy, just enough to avoid straining the back. Breathe in.

Next

Exhale while flattening and lifting your abs to initiate a smooth lift. Everything should be in harmony – your head, ribcage, arms and legs – as if they are a single unit making a 'C' shape from the tips of your toes to the tips of your fingers. The centre of your back and your hips should remain firmly in place and your legs steady. The movement comes from your abs pulling your chest up and forward.

Return to the starting position. Do 4 reps to start, gradually increasing to two sets of 8–16.

After each curl workout go to page 75 for your cool-down exercises

Nicki Waterman's Flat Stomach Plan

Super abs routine

For the very fit and experienced, here is a powerful three-in-one routine that will work the entire gamut of your ab muscles. For best results, work through all three, without resting in between.

Always warm up and stretch first before any workout session

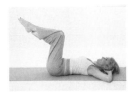

Stretch up and Reach

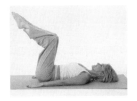

High Reverse Curl

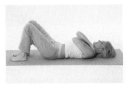 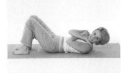

Twisting Curl

Stretch Up and Reach

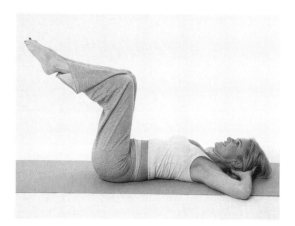 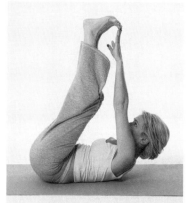

Tips:
Looking along your arms to the tips of your fingers as you lift will help keep your head in the correct position. Lower your knees towards your torso when you return to the starting position each time.

Begin
Lie on the floor, in the basic starting position, head cradled in hands. Now raise your legs so that your knees are bent and over your hips and your lower legs are slightly elevated. This should be comfortable – if you feel any strain on your back, try bending the knees slightly more. Keep your hips and lower back on the floor throughout. Inhale deeply.

Next
Exhale as you lift, stretching both arms towards your feet. At the same time straighten your knees and push the feet up towards the ceiling, keeping them flat, not pointed. The effort in the lift must come from the long abdominal (tummy) muscles bringing the ribcage and pubic area closer together.

Return to the starting position and repeat. Do 4–8 reps, gradually increasing to two sets of 8–16.

Don't stop! Continue straight on with ...

Nicki Waterman's Flat Stomach Plan

High Reverse Curl

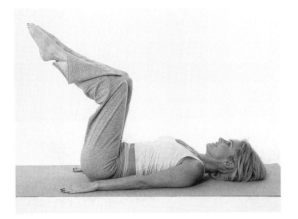 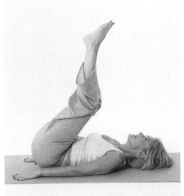

Tips:

Maintain the compression of the abs throughout the entire hips lift. Don't come down with a crash or let your knees flop down onto your chest.

Begin

Lie on your back on the floor with your arms straight and at a comfortable angle a few inches from your body, palms flat down to provide a little balance and support. Your knees should be bent over your hips with your back and pelvis pressed to the floor. Breathe in.

Next

Start to exhale and contract your abs, lifting your hips as high as possible in a reverse curl, then slowly straighten your legs. Your feet should end up leaning towards and over your chest. Your head and upper back will still be on the floor. Hold then smoothly uncurl.

Do 4–8 reps, gradually increasing to two sets of 8–16.

Again, don't stop. Continue straight on with ...

Twisting Curl

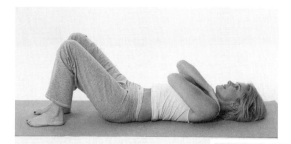

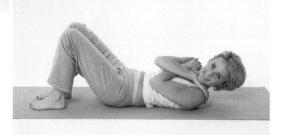

Tip:
The twist must come from the contraction of the obliques at your waist, not by leading from your shoulders.

Begin
Lie in the basic position on your back with your knees up, feet hip-width apart and at a comfortable distance from your buttocks. Fold your arms across your chest, hands on opposite shoulders. Breathe in.

Next
Exhale as you compress your abs in and up. Curl your upper back smoothly up towards your knees and as you do so twist your body to the left. Hold then reverse back to start.

Repeat towards the right. Do 4–8 reps, gradually increasing to two sets of 8–16.

After each curl workout go to page 75 for your cool-down exercises

Nicki Waterman's Flat Stomach Plan

CHAPTER SEVEN

Cool Down and Relax

During your ab routine you focused on tightening your tummy muscles, on pulling them in hard towards your back and up into your ribcage. Now it's time to cool down and relax. However, that doesn't mean you can just flop into a chair in relief.

After your ab workout (indeed, after any form of hard exercise) you need to focus on stretching and relaxing. This minimizes soreness in the muscles and helps prevent injury from cramp or strain. Stretching and relaxing gently while your body is still hot will increase flexibility and make you feel even better. Then, afterwards, a warm shower, a change of clothing and you'll feel – and look – a million dollars.

You will find that many of these cooling-down stretches are the same as those featured in the warming-up section since the purpose is to gently stretch the same muscles at the start and finish of your curl session. They are shown again here to prevent you having to flick back and forth between sections.

Hold each stretch for at least 30 counts

The Neck Stretch

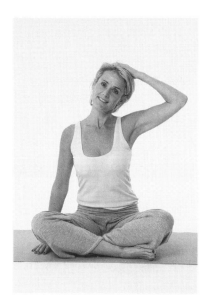

Begin

Sit on the floor, as tall as you can, with your legs loosely crossed. Place an open hand on the crown of your head and rest the other hand on the floor.

Next

Applying gentle pressure with your hand, lower your left ear towards your left shoulder. At the same time, push your shoulder downwards. Hold then relax.

Repeat on the other side.

Nicki Waterman's Flat Stomach Plan

Sit Up and Stretch

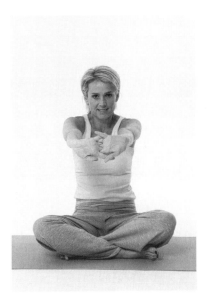

Begin

Sit on the ground, legs loosely crossed, as tall as you can. With shoulders relaxed, raise your arms, interlocking your fingers above your head, palms facing forward.

Next

To stretch your back, remain tall in the body while you bring your arms down and forward, curving your back forward. At the same time, draw your abs in and up into your ribcage. Hold, then reverse back to the starting position, arms above head, sitting up nice and tall.

Curl Up and Stretch

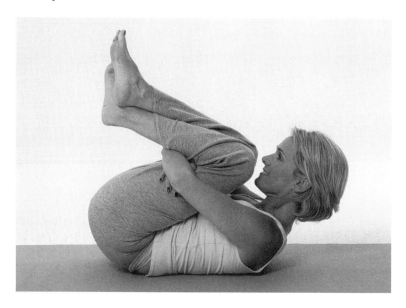

Begin

Lie on your back as you would for a basic curl, knees raised, feet on the floor. Now clasp your hands together behind your knees and bring your knees up towards your chest.

Next

Now imagine that you are a hedgehog. Exhale while smoothly coming up as if into a curl, bringing your head and shoulders close to your knees. Your back should feel stretched. Hold then relax.

Floor Twist and Stretch

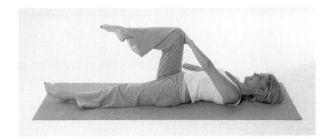

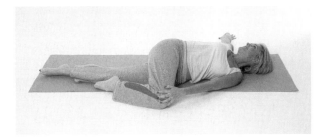

Begin

Lie full length and relaxed on the floor, your arms loosely outstretched for balance in the move. Lift your right knee up partly towards your chest and place your left hand on the outside of your right thigh just above the knee.

Next

Keeping both shoulders and upper back down against the floor as much as possible, use your left hand to bring your right knee across your body towards the opposite side. You will feel your hip muscle stretching. Now push that knee even further down towards the floor, allowing your right shoulder to move up off the floor only as much as necessary. Feel that long stretch expanding into your lower back. Hold then relax.

Repeat on the other side.

Lunge Stretch

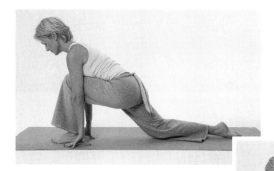

Begin

Kneel down on the floor. Now, ensuring that your head, neck, shoulders and back are all aligned correctly with your back – step forward and lean over your left knee. Your chest must remain lifted – don't sag in the middle or allow your head to droop. Your arms should be straight down on either side of your left foot, fingertips resting on the floor.

Next

Holding your torso up, lunge forward slowly onto your left leg, making sure that the knee remains directly above your ankle. You should feel the front thigh muscles of the right leg stretch. Hold then relax.

Repeat on the other side.

Stand Up and Stretch

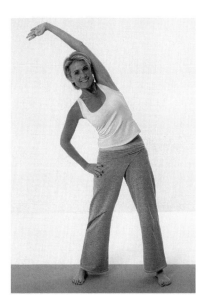

Begin
Stand upright, your back stretched and tall, your legs hip-width apart. Bend your knees just a little and put your left hand on your left thigh, reaching up with the right arm above your shoulder. Your head, neck and shoulders should be in their correct basic position.

Next
Slowly stretch over to your left side, your right arm still held up. You'll feel your waist stretching. Hold then relax.

Repeat on the other side.

Stand Up and Curl

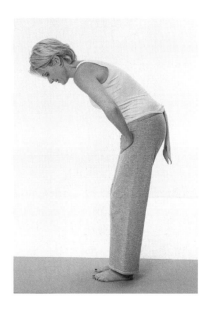

Begin
Stand upright, legs hip-width apart and your hands on the top of your thighs. Now lean over slightly from the hips, bending the knees a little – but don't sag. Make sure that your head, neck, shoulders and back are all aligned and straight and your chest is lifted.

Next
Pull your tummy in as far as you can while continuing to keep your chest up and your head and back aligned. You should feel the stretch in your back. Hold then relax.

Shoulder Back Pull

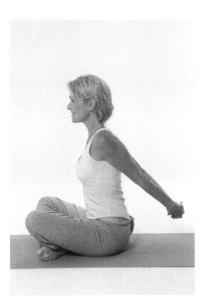

This final stretch is a great cooling-down exercise that helps your shoulder muscles to stretch and relax and gives you an overall feeling of well-being.

Begin

Sit upright, nice and straight, tummy tucked in and flat, your legs crossed loosely. Put your arms behind your buttocks, your hands clasped and loosely resting on the floor. Already you should feel your shoulders stretching and expanding your chest.

Next

Still maintaining your nice upright posture, lift your hands back, up and away from you as far as they will reach, until you feel some tension in your shoulders. Keeping your arms straight, hold until you feel some easing of the tension, then raise a little more to another degree of tension. Hold. The pattern should be tension and ease, tension and ease. Hold then relax.

CHAPTER EIGHT

Preventing Back Problems

Back pain is an incredibly commonplace problem among people of all ages, and one of the leading causes of back pain is bad posture. Poor postural habits can ultimately result in a deterioration of the structures of the spinal column, including the discs. The discs – soft, spongy 'cushions' filled with viscous fluid – lie between each vertebra of the spine and are responsible for protecting the spinal cord from everyday impact activities (walking, running, jumping etc.) and for allowing great flexibility of movement (such as bending backwards, forwards and sideways and rotating the torso).

In order to carry out these functions, the discs and the spine in general must be supported by strong back muscles. However, instead of strengthening these muscles, many people inflict damage on their back by ignoring them. They sit slumped over a desk for long periods with shoulders and back rounded, or they stand lopsided – one hip stuck forward, the pelvic girdle on a slope and their back twisted. They watch television for hours on end in a seat that doesn't support the back, or sleep in a bed that has an overly soft mattress. All these everyday activities and many more – habitually carrying a heavy bag on the same shoulder, carrying a baby awkwardly, bending, digging and so on – can have a detrimental effect on the back.

In addition to contorting the structures of the back by bad everyday posture, further damage is inflicted simply by a lack of exercise. This leads to the torso and back muscles losing strength and slackening, with a resultant strain on the spine. Note how babies and toddlers, who are constantly active, are always fit and supple. This is what we lose as we age – if we do not ensure that our back and abdominal (tummy) muscles are strong and flexible enough to support the spine.

Being overweight can also strain the back. Poor posture coupled with awkward, jerky movement while exercising or lifting puts an uneven strain on the discs. Arching and rounding the back, perhaps while seated or lying awkwardly or bending too quickly and lifting, changes the angle of pressure on the discs. If the back muscles aren't strong or flexible enough to support the spine and allow a wide range of movement, in time the discs can protrude, or rupture – and the result of this is inevitably immobility and pain.

Most people know all this, yet they still continue with their bad habits until something drastic happens, such as a slipped disc.

So what is the solution?

Good posture largely depends on having strong back and abdominal (tummy) muscles to hold the spine, neck, head and the hips in proper alignment and to allow great flexibility of movement.

In order to achieve this, the muscles in the front and back of the body work in opposition to each other. Their structure is also different. The abdominals are the same length and stretch from the ribcage to the pelvic girdle, like a cradle that holds and protects the vital organs. The back muscles vary a great deal in length. Some are very long and extend the full length of the back while others run from one vertebra to another and are extremely short. The long muscles provide flexibility while the short ones are far more inflexible – after all, their job is to hold the spine in place so that we can stand upright without too much flexion putting an uneven strain on the discs. However, the correct stretching exercises can add to spinal flexibility.

There is a wide range of exercises to help strengthen the abdominals and the back. And, as this book demonstrates, the best exercises for the lower back and abdominal muscles are curls. Curls undoubtedly help to strengthen, tone and give flexibility to the tummy muscles, as well as stretching and strengthening both the long and short back muscles. In this section you will find exercises specifically designed for the back. It is important to follow them carefully, working in a smooth, controlled way to help ensure that all the muscles are correctly worked and the spine and discs are protected from damage. Fast, uneven and jerky movements will not only be ineffective but could lead to a lower back injury.

Try to do at least three of these back-strengthening exercises after your curl session. If you have time for only one, make it The Cat. It is a very simple and safe exercise that stretches and strengthens the back, so it is perfect for anyone with a tight or stiff back. Don't rush into a large number of these back exercises on the basis that more is better. *They are not a cure, but a preventative*. Take it easy at first, do just a few repetitions and as soon as you feel any strain, stop.

Always finish with the back cool-down exercises (see pages 93–5) in addition to your regular cooling-down routine.

If you already suffer from existing back pain or any back-related problems, check with your doctor or physiotherapist before doing these exercises. I repeat – these exercises are not a cure but a means of helping prevent problems.

Back strengthening exercises
The Cat

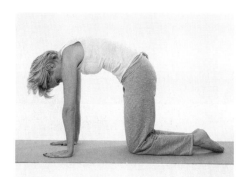 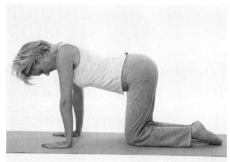

Begin

Get down on your hands and knees, with your arms below your shoulders and your knees hip-width apart directly under your hips. Keeping your back straight and level, with your head and neck in alignment, pull your abs in and up.

Next

Using your tummy muscles, fully round your spine upwards as far you can go without moving the position of your legs or arms. Do this slowly then hold for a count of 10. As your back becomes stronger, gradually increase the count to 20–30.

Now curve your spine in the opposite, concave direction towards the floor. Still keeping your legs and arms vertical and in the same position, arch your neck, head and buttocks upwards as high as they will comfortably go. Don't force it. Hold for a count of four then release. As you gain in strength, you can gradually hold for longer.

Return to the start position and relax for a moment or two before standing up.

Swimmer's Stretch

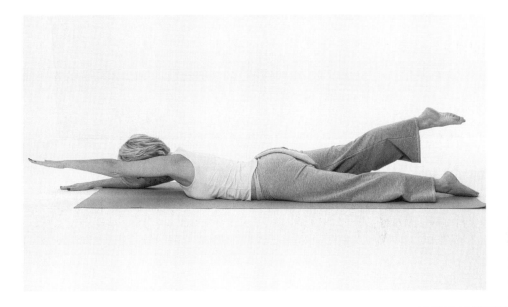

Begin

Lie face down on the floor with feet and arms pointing in opposite directions. Lift your tummy in and up, but keep your hips pressed down.

Next

Still keeping your tummy lifted, stretch out your left arm and your right leg. You should find they lift up horizontally from the floor, but ensure that your hips remain pressed down. If it makes it more comfortable, turn your head towards the arm you are lifting, but keep your neck relaxed and aligned with your spine.

Now return your arm and leg to the floor and do 8–10 reps. Gradually increase this to two sets of 8–10. Repeat with the right arm and the left leg.

Hyper Extensions

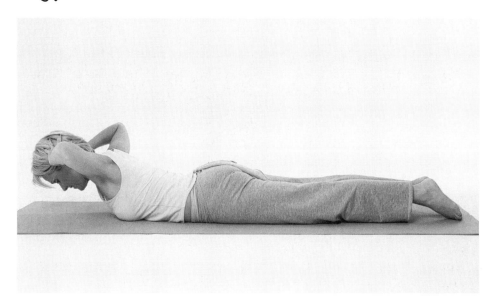

Begin

Lie face down on the floor with your hands on the back of your head. Your fingers should be open but they don't need to meet. Your legs should be together and firmly pressed on the floor, feet stretched.

Next

Now try to lengthen your body and, as you do so, your upper body will *slowly* lift. The aim is not to lift your head as high as it will go, but to allow the movement to come from the contraction of your back muscles. Remember to keep your hips pressed down and your head and neck aligned.

Relax back into the starting position and repeat, doing 4 reps. Gradually increase the number of reps as your back becomes stronger. This is a hard exercise so don't force it. If you have difficulty with lifting or your movements are at all jerky, stop until your back is stronger.

Nicki Waterman's Flat Stomach Plan

Opposite Arm and Leg Balance

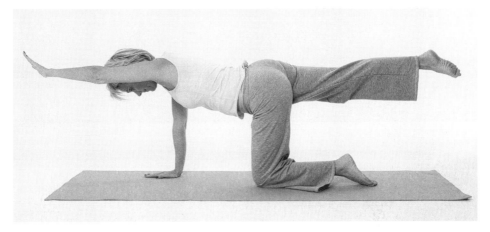

Tip:
To ensure that you hold your back flat and don't arch your spine or jerk your buttocks or head up, balance your weight evenly between the supporting hand and leg.

This exercise strengthens the back and improves balance. It is not easy and you will find that you are fighting gravity to keep your body level.

Begin
Kneel on your hands and knees on the floor, your arms in a straight line below your shoulders and your legs hip-width apart, with your knees directly under your hips. Make sure your back is flat and your head and neck are properly aligned.

Next
Using your tummy muscles to hold your hips and lower back firmly in place, *slowly* extend your left arm and your right leg until they are straight out and horizontal to the floor. Do not raise them so much that you get into a swayback (concave) position. In order to keep your head level it will help if you look down.

Hold for a count of four then release and return to the starting position. Repeat once more. Gradually build up to 8 reps, holding each for a count of four.

Repeat with the right arm and left leg, making sure that you do an equal number of reps on each side.

Forearm Press

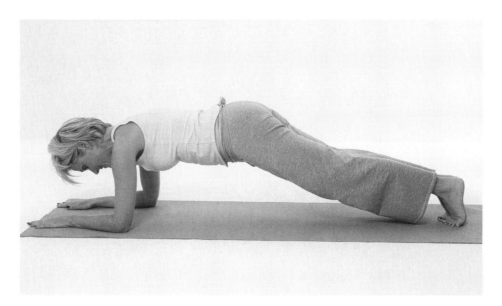

Begin

Kneel down on the floor, palms flat and your weight resting on your forearms. Your legs should be together, knees directly below your hips. Move onto the balls of your feet and raise your heels. Your back should be straight, with your head and neck in their natural alignment. Pull your abs in and up.

Next

With your weight evenly distributed on your forearms, and keeping your back flat, use your abs to help you lift as you slowly straighten your legs. Keep your neck in its natural position – don't lift your head or let it flop down. Hold for a count of four then slowly relax your knees back to their original position.

Repeat once more. Gradually work up to 8 reps, holding each one for a count of four.

Your back cool-down exercises now follow on

Nicki Waterman's Flat Stomach Plan

Cool down exercises for the back

Curl Up and Stretch

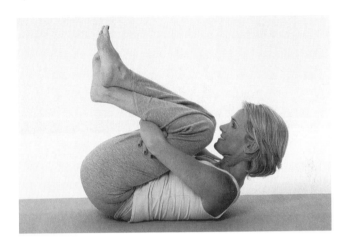

Begin
Lie on your back as you would for a basic curl, knees raised, feet on the floor. Clasp your hands together behind your knees and bring your knees up towards your chest.

Next
Now imagine that you are a hedgehog. Exhale while smoothly coming up as if into a curl, bringing your head and shoulders close to your knees. Your back should feel stretched. Hold then relax.

Twist and Stretch

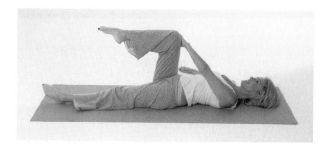

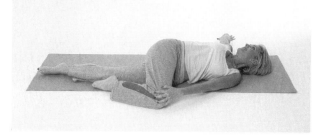

Begin

Lie full length and relaxed on the floor, your arms loosely outstretched for balance in the move. Lift your right knee up partly towards your chest and place your left hand on the outside of your right thigh just above the knee.

Next

Keeping both shoulders and upper back down against the floor as much as possible, use your left hand to bring your right knee across your body towards the opposite side. You will feel your hip muscle stretching. Now push that knee even further down towards the floor, allowing your right shoulder to move up off the floor only as much as necessary. Feel that long stretch expanding into your lower back. Hold then relax.

Repeat on the other side.

The Neck Stretch

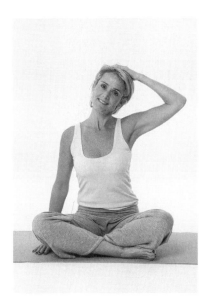

Begin

Sit on the ground, as tall as you can, legs loosely crossed. Place one hand on the crown of your head and rest the other hand on the floor.

Next

Applying gentle pressure with your hand, lower your left ear towards your left shoulder. At the same time, push your shoulder downwards. Hold then relax.

Repeat on the other side.

CHAPTER NINE

Exercise and Pregnancy

Gentle curls during pregnancy

A web of strong abdominal and back muscles is a great bonus for a pregnant woman, as they help support the extra weight of the baby – especially as the months pass and the strain grows greater. Ideally, then, you should already be in peak condition when you become pregnant.

If you have been working out, there is no reason why you should stop when you become pregnant (there are some rare exceptions to this, so do of course seek your doctor's advice first). Although you should be aware that there can be some medical problems connected with strenuous exercise during pregnancy, working out sensibly (again, seek your doctor's advice on what is sensible for you) should not be a problem. In fact, working out in a controlled and gentle way is highly recommended for the mum-to-be. The American College of Obstetricians and Gynecologists recently stated that pregnant women should engage in 30 minutes or more of moderate exercise five days a week. And remember, it is not only beneficial for the mother – exercise ensures that plenty of oxygen-rich blood reaches the developing embryo.

As you go into the fourth month of pregnancy you should alter the focus of your routine from strength training to stretches that encourage flexibility. You should also reduce the number of reps. Choose exercises that allow you to sit – preferably with back support – instead of standing (to avoid balance problems), and don't leap up and down in hard impact moves. Most experts also advise against lying on your back due to the pressure on the vena cava, the muscle that returns blood from the lower body to the heart. Doing most of your usual curls after your belly rises above the pubic bone is also cautioned against since the stress can be a factor in abdominal (tummy muscle) separation (see Diastasis, below). If you are worried about doing your usual exercise at this stage, why not try gentle belly dancing (see page 127) The movements of dancing strengthen the abs with very little strain and will also help during labour.

For those who feel able to continue with a modified ab routine, try a supported curl, propping up your head and shoulders with pillows or a Swiss Ball. In addition, doing a few moderate stretches each day is a good idea as this will help relieve pressure on your lower back. Do bear in mind, however, that the hormone relaxin, which is produced during pregnancy, loosens the joints so you will be more prone to pulls and injuries. It is important, therefore, to limit your range of motion and keep your movements slow and controlled.

The following two exercises and the pelvic floor exercises on page 102 are suitable during pregnancy.

Diastasis

Diastasis, or separation, occurs when the two halves of the long rectus abdominus muscle in the middle of your belly separate during pregnancy. You can check for this yourself. Lie on your back with your knees bent. (If you start to feel faint while on your back, roll to your left side and use pillows under your shoulder to prop yourself up.) Now put your fingertips 3–5cm (1–2in) below your belly button, fingers facing downwards. Lift your head as high as you can. If you feel a ridge protruding from the midline of your tummy, or if you can put more than one or two fingers in between the muscles, you'll know you have separation. The condition isn't painful and will not harm the baby, but it is important if you have it to take extra care when exercising. Try a modified ab curl.

Rock and Back Arch

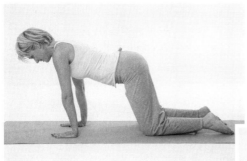

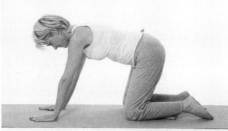

Begin

Kneel on the floor on all fours, with your arms straight below your shoulders, palms face down. Your legs should be hip-width apart, knees directly below your hips.

Next

Now rock gently back and forth while you count to five. Return to the original position and gently arch your back. Keep your hips down and your head and neck correctly aligned. Repeat five times. Try to find time to do this several times a day.

Modified Ab Curl

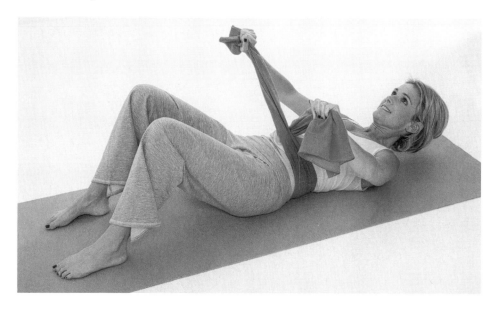

Begin

Fold a sheet or a sarong lengthways to about 20cm (8in) wide, wrap it around your waist from the back and crisscross it in front. Don't knot it. Now lie on your back in the basic curl position with knees bent. (If you are past the first month, prop yourself up with pillows so that your shoulders are higher than your belly.)

Next

Grasp and pull the ends of the sheet up and outwards at 45-degree angles as you *gently* contract your tummy muscles. Exhale and raise your head. Do not lift your shoulders.

Here's another method of doing a supported curl, using your arms instead of a sheet or sarong:

Lie on your back with your knees bent, shoulders supported on pillows if necessary. Now cross your arms across your tummy, squeezing the muscles together as you exhale. Gently contract the abs, lifting only your head (not your shoulders). Stop at once if you feel faint or experience any discomfort.

Nicki Waterman's Flat Stomach Plan

The importance of the pelvic floor muscles

You've probably never given them a second thought before, but during pregnancy and childbirth your pelvic floor muscles really come into their own. They support everything in your pelvis, including your uterus, bladder and bowel. Your health and comfort are greatly affected by the ability of the pelvic muscles to do their job.

During pregnancy the extra weight of your baby, the amniotic fluid and the womb put a greater burden on your pelvic floor. You can tell if it's coping with this strain when you sneeze or jump up and down – if there is a leakage of urine, your muscles aren't strong enough.

It is particularly important that your pelvic floor is in good shape when you give birth. You release these muscles as you bear down in the final stages, and they are stretched as your baby is delivered. If your pelvic floor is in good condition then it will return to its normal state much quicker after the birth. If it is not, you could end up experiencing problems with stress incontinence. (Keeping your pelvic floor muscles in shape is just as important when you're not pregnant – it can even enhance your sex life. Squeezing your pelvic floor during intercourse makes it more pleasurable for you and your partner.)

By practising a few quick and easy pelvic floor exercises every day you can have a more comfortable pregnancy, an easier delivery and a quicker recovery. It's all about muscle tone – the more toned and flexible your pelvic floor, the better it will cope.

Pelvic floor exercises

Before you start these exercises, you need to know which are your pelvic floor muscles. To do this, imagine peeing and stopping mid-flow. The muscles you use to do this make up your pelvic floor. Do both the following exercises six times a day.

Exercise 1

Sit upright in a comfortable chair. Concentrate on your pelvic floor and relax the rest of your body. Tense your pelvic floor and hold it until the muscles start to feel tired and begin to tremble. Try to hold for a count of at least 10 or 15. Release them slowly, breathing out as you do so. Repeat this exercise 10 times. This will help to build strength in the muscles and the exercise will become easier with practice.

Exercise 2

Concentrate on your pelvic floor and relax the rest of your body. Tense your pelvic floor and do 10 quick tense-and-release cycles, without holding for a count. This will help to build muscle tone.

Post-natal exercises

A number of women experience trouble bringing their tummy back to its original tone and size after childbirth. When you consider that it has taken nine months for the stomach to stretch to hold your baby, you will appreciate that afterwards, gentle but steady perseverance is the key to trimming those inches away and tightening stretched muscles. For most women, a combination of time and abdominal exercises should help the tummy return to its original size.

It is important that you regain the strength of your ab muscles after the birth of your baby, as strong muscles help prevent lower back injury – as well as helping you regain a flat stomach. Check with your doctor when you can begin exercising again. Do be aware, however, that you are unlikely to be able to work at the same pace or with the same amount of energy every day as you normally would have done pre-pregnancy. If being pregnant is tiring, many women swear that 'life after baby' can be downright exhausting. Some days, you just won't feel like working out – especially if you've been up all night. Don't force the pace at such times – do some easy exercises, or take a walk with the baby. However, some perseverance is necessary if you're going to get rid of that stretched tummy, so don't let more than a couple of days pass before you're back with your routine to beat that bump.

The following exercises are in order of difficulty, so work through them gradually as your ability to do them increases. Obviously, if you feel any pain or discomfort stop.

Don't forget to warm up before exercising and to cool down afterwards

Bridging

Begin

Lie on your back with your knees bent, feet flat on the floor and your hands on your tummy. Keep a small 'natural' curve in your lower back. Tilt your pelvis so that your pubic bone lifts up and your lower back presses into the floor. Slowly peel your lower back off the floor and continue through your mid-back and up into the ribcage. Try to press each vertebra down into the floor before peeling off. Continue to lift until the tips of your shoulder blades are just off the floor, but make sure you don't lift onto your neck. Pause.

Next

Keeping your buttocks lifted, lower with control, using your tummy muscles to press each of the vertebrae back into the floor. You will find some sections of your back feel stiffer than others. Concentrate on these less mobile areas by slowing down the movement to ease out tension and lengthen your spine further.

Repeat 8 times.

Abdominal Hollowing

Begin

Lie on your back with your knees bent, feet flat on the floor and your hands resting on your tummy. Keep a small 'natural' curve in your lower back. Breathe in.

Next

As you breathe out, draw in your tummy muscles and concentrate on pulling your navel down away from your hands and towards your spine. Release as you breathe in without letting your tummy swell.

Repeat 8–10 times.

Pelvic Tilt

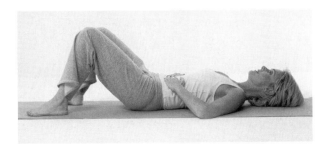

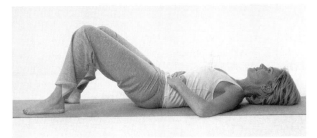

Begin

Lie on your back with your knees bent, feet flat on the floor. Place your hands on your stomach so that you can feel the tightening muscles.

Next

Gently tighten your stomach muscles and push the arch of your back towards the floor. Squeeze your bottom tight. Hold the position for 20 seconds and relax.

Repeat 8–10 times.

Ab Curl

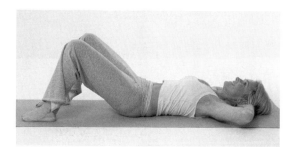

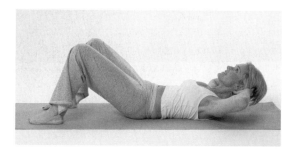

Tip:

If you feel your stomach protruding during the curl, stop. Make a conscious effort to pull it in and up and then continue with the exercise. The purpose of a curl is to train your stomach to be flat.

Begin

Lie on your back with your knees bent, feet flat on the floor and hip-width apart. With elbows on the floor at right angles to your head, cradle your head in your hands. Inhale deeply and prepare to lift.

Next

Exhale, pulling your tummy in and up. This will start to smoothly lift your shoulders and ribcage off the floor. Keep your shoulders back and relaxed, head cradled in hands, elbows and arms still level and at right angles to your head. Don't strain or try to sit up. Go as far up as is comfortable while keeping your tummy flat and your lower spine pressed against the floor. Your feet should not move.

Repeat 8–10 times.

Nicki Waterman's Flat Stomach Plan

Cross and Curl

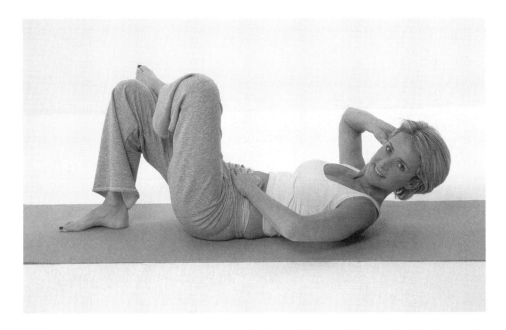

Begin

Lie on your back with your knees bent, feet flat on the floor. Bring one leg up and place the ankle on the opposite thigh just above the knee. Rest your head in the opposite hand to the raised leg and lay your other hand flat on your tummy, fingers spread. Let both elbows rest on the ground to start. Breathe in deeply.

Next

Let your breath out smoothly as you come up into the curl and, as you do so, start to twist by lifting and rotating the shoulder of the arm supporting the head, and your ribcage, towards the raised knee. Don't swing your elbow forward or you will find that you are pulling on your neck.

Repeat 7–9 times, doing an equal number of reps on both sides.

Elbow to the Floor

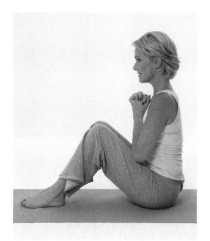

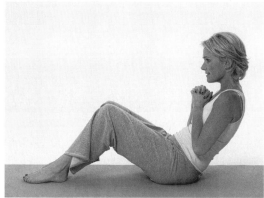

Begin
Sit on the floor, knees bent and hands together in front of you.

Next
Slowly lean backwards, pressing each elbow towards the floor, then gradually work back to your starting position.
Do 8–10 reps then repeat.

Reach Your Toes

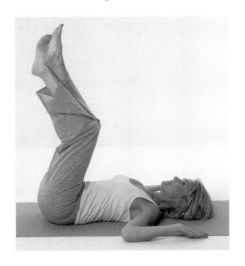

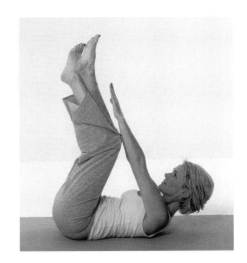

Begin
Lie on the floor with your hands just above your shoulders and bend your hips so your legs are vertical and crossed at the ankles.

Next
Lift your head and shoulders off the floor, gently reach up towards your toes then return to the starting position.

Do 8–10 reps then repeat.

Reverse Curl

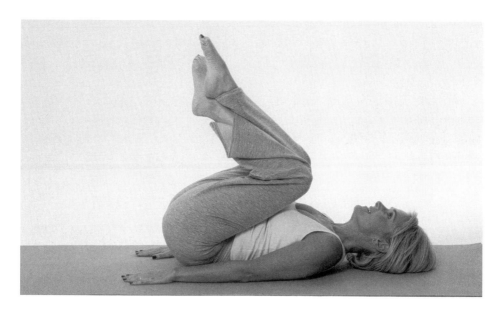

Begin

Lie flat, with knees up and bent as close to your chest as possible, calves resting on your thighs, ankles crossed. Your arms should be lying on the floor along your sides, palms facing down so you can push *gently* if necessary.

Next

Breathe in deeply. Now exhale, at the same time pressing your tummy in and up towards your ribcage while starting to gradually curl up the lower part of your spine. You should feel your pelvis move up towards your ribcage. Concentrate on curling the spine using the tummy muscles to pull your knees forward and not your leg muscles.

Return to the starting position by smoothly uncurling your spine, letting your tailbone down towards the floor. (Obviously it won't completely touch the floor because your knees are up.) Start with 4 reps, building up to 8–10.

Warrior Curl

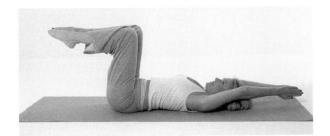

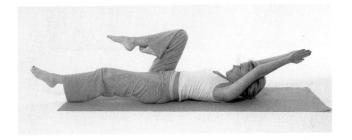

Begin

Lie on your back with your arms extended behind your head, palms together. Bend your knees and place your feet flat on the floor, hip-width apart. Still keeping your arms behind you, lift them a few inches above the floor. At the same time, bring your knees up directly over your hips, keeping your lower legs parallel to the floor. Pull your abs in and up as you inhale.

Next

Exhale as you bring your right knee towards your body and extend your left leg straight out. Stretch as you continue to pull the abs in and up. Repeat, straightening the opposite leg.

Do 6 reps to start with, increasing to 20 as your stomach gets stronger.

Prayers

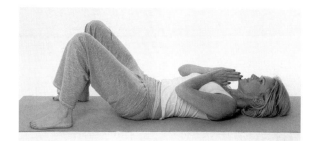

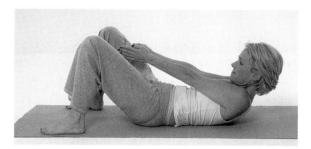

Begin

Lie on your back with your knees bent, feet flat on the floor 12cm (5in) further out than hip-width apart. Put your palms together over your chest. Pull your abs in tight and up. Inhale.

Next

Drop your chin slightly to support your head. With your palms still together, reach forward between your thighs as you exhale, simultaneously curling smoothly forward, 12cm (5in) off the floor. Hold.

Uncurl slowly, without letting the top of your back touch the floor. Keep your shoulders relaxed and back and your head and neck properly aligned.

Repeat 5 times, gradually building up to 20 reps.

Once you have reached this stage you can try the Curl-free Workout (see pages 121–126). The routine is inspired by various forms of exercise – such as yoga, Pilates and kick-boxing – and is great for really honing those abs muscles

Yoga for two

Millions of women practice yoga not only for its physical benefits – firmer abs, sleeker arms, tighter butt – but also to recharge emotionally. What better way to shape-up while de-stressing? The yoga exercises here have an added bonus – each can be done with your baby and it's a great way of bonding. Feel free to sing to your baby, talk, act silly – whatever seems natural. Do this routine three or four times a week for total body toning and relaxation. (All new mums should check with their doctor before doing any workout.)

Don't forget to warm up before exercising and to cool down afterwards

Boat Pose

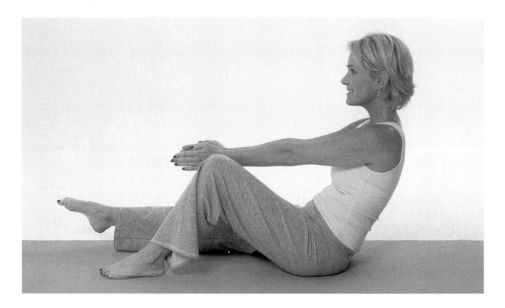

This exercise strengthens the tummy muscles, back, shoulders and legs.

Begin

Sit on the floor with your knees bent and your feet flat on the floor, with your baby facing you on your lap. Lean back slightly, exhale and straighten the lower part of one leg, keeping the foot of the other leg on the floor.

Inhale, extending both arms in front at about knee height (or hold on to your baby with one arm), balancing on the 'sitting bones' of your bottom. Repeat, straightening the other leg.

Next

For an added challenge, try extending both legs at the same time. Hold here and sing a chorus of 'Row, Row, Row Your Boat' to your baby, rowing with your arms. At the last part of the chorus, straighten and lower both legs to floor, keeping your baby on your lap. Now go directly into the Forward Bend.

Nicki Waterman's Flat Stomach Plan

Forward Bend

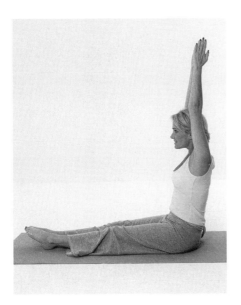 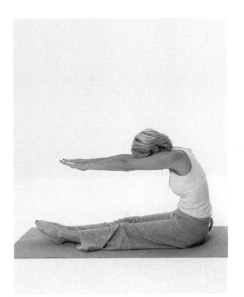

A forward bend stretches the back, hamstrings (backs of thighs) and shoulders, and tones the tummy muscles. Depending on your flexibility, you can do all sorts of playful things with your baby in this position, such as blowing on his or her belly.

Begin

Sit with your legs extended forward and your baby cradled between your thighs or calves. Sit up tall. Inhale and lift both arms out to the sides and above your head, palms facing in.

Next

Exhale while lowering your arms, palms facing down. Repeat 3 or 4 times. On the last exhalation, bend forward from your hips toward your baby. Stay in this position for about 10 full breaths and play with your baby (kiss their tummy, stroke their face, hold hands etc.).

Combined Cat and Child's Pose

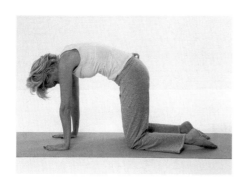

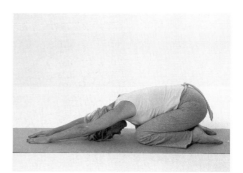

This is great for stretching the back, shoulders and chest, and toning the arms and tummy muscles. It's a useful pose both during and after pregnancy because it relieves pressure on the lower back and shoulders.

Begin

Start on all fours with your baby in front of you on a blanket. Your hands should be under your shoulders at about the same level as your baby's belly button. Inhale, lift your chin and tailbone up and arch your spine.

Next

Exhale and round your spine, squeezing your abs in while moving your head and tailbone down. Gaze at your baby, making eye contact. Repeat 3 or 4 times. On the last repetition, move your tailbone back toward your heels, chest on thighs, knees slightly apart and arms extended in front of your body (child's pose). Feel the stretch in your shoulders and back. Hold for a few counts, then go into the Downward Dog pose.

Downward Dog

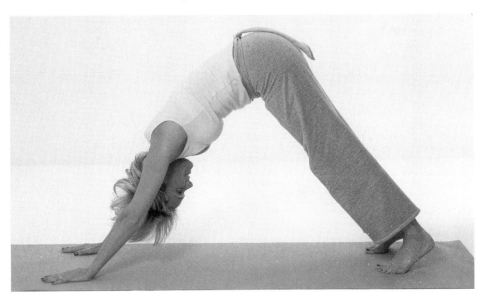

This stretches the legs, back and shoulders, as well as strengthening the arms, chest and tummy muscles.

Begin

From the Child's Pose return to all fours, then curl your toes under and press your heels down.

Next

Straighten your legs, lifting your tailbone toward the ceiling until you're in an inverted V position (your baby will still be on the floor below you). If necessary, keep your knees slightly bent, then slowly straighten one leg at a time, moving your heels towards the floor. Pull your shoulders back, lengthening your back, and make funny faces and noises. Hold for as long as is comfortable.

Backbend

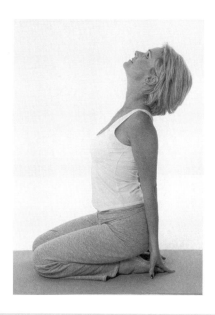
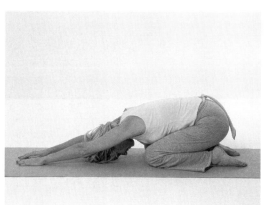

Feeding or holding your baby requires you to constantly lean forward, which rounds the shoulders and overextends the upper back. This pose is a great way to counterbalance that action. It stretches the chest, shoulders and tummy muscles, and improves posture.

Begin

Sit on your heels, legs hip-distance apart, tops of feet on the floor. Inhaling, lift your hips up and lengthen your thighs. Exhale, arch your back, bring your chest towards the ceiling and let your head gently drop back. Bring your hands towards your heels for support (or out to sides for a greater challenge). Inhale and straighten your spine.

Next

Move back into the Child's Pose: bring your chest to your thighs and sit on your heels while looking at your baby. Repeat the pose 5 times.

Nicki Waterman's Flat Stomach Plan

Seated Twist

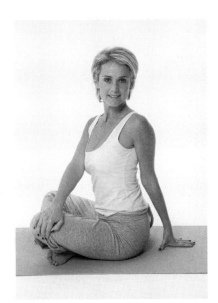

This pose stretches the back, neck and tummy muscles.

Begin

Sit cross-legged on the floor with your baby on your lap. Exhale and bring your left hand to your right knee while keeping your right hand behind you for support. Inhale and lengthen your spine by sitting as tall and high on your sitting bones as you can.

Next

Exhale and slowly twist to the right, starting at the base of your spine and moving upward through the naval, ribs, chest, shoulders, neck and, finally, head. Hold for 2 or 3 deep, relaxing breaths. Repeat, twisting in the opposite direction.

CHAPTER TEN

The Curl-Free Workout

Varying your workout routine with some different moves will prevent boredom, challenge your body – and is fun. Just to add a little spice, try these alternative exercises for a firm, flat stomach. My curl-free workout is based on hard-hitting moves from Pilates, yoga, gymnastics and boxing. The idea is to create leaner, stronger muscles that define your abs and waist. Exercise on its own will also burn up calories and help you to lose weight – but if you watch what you eat as well, then you will reach that goal of a new, defined you much more quickly – and when you look good, you feel better too.

Exchange this curl-free routine for your normal abs workout two or three times a week, performing three sets (beginners can start with two) of 8 to 18 repetitions per move. Keep your abs contracted during the moves and rest for just 20 seconds in between if necessary. The breathing routine that you learned on page 16 should be followed throughout.

Don't forget to warm up before exercising and to cool down afterwards

Side-Lying Lift

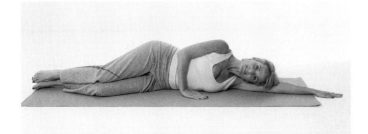

Tip:
In this exercise you must resist the temptation to use your arms to help you lift.

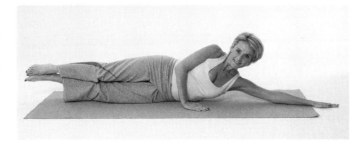

This exercise is based on Pilates (the exercise method developed many years ago by Joseph H. Pilates). It targets the large tummy muscles that run from the ribcage to the pubic bone and obliquely through the waist.

Begin
Lie on your left side, hips and legs stacked, feet together and left arm extended on the floor in line with your body, palm down. Keep your head and neck lifted but relaxed. Bring your right hand in front of your chest for support and balance, elbow slightly bent, palm resting on the floor.

Next
Exhale and contract your abs. Now, using the power of your middle, slowly lift your legs and upper body 5–10cm (2–4in), then slowly release. Don't roll back.

Start with two sets of 8 reps, working up to three sets of 18. Repeat on the other side, making sure you do the same number of reps on each side.

The Star Stretch

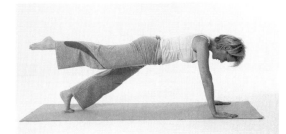

Tip:
Don't hump up your back – think long, lean and stretched.

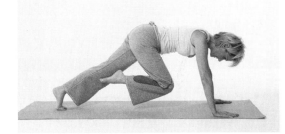

Developed from yoga and Pilates, this exercise targets all the lower abs, but in particular the muscles below the navel.

Begin

Lie stretched out, face down on the floor and push yourself up onto the palms of your hands and your toes, keeping your body in a straight line. (Your head must be aligned with shoulders, chest in line with hips. Your arms will be straight, elbows below your shoulders.) Focus your eyes on the floor.

Next

Shift your body weight back onto your feet so your arms don't bear all your weight. Keeping your abs tight, point your right foot as you lift your right leg to hip height. Hold just until you find your balance.

Keeping your abs tight, bring your right knee forward towards your arm until that knee is pointing toward the floor. Hold for 5 seconds before straightening your leg. Lower your leg towards the floor, keeping the toes pointed and stretched.

Do two lots of 8 reps to start, working up to three sets of 8–18. Switch to opposite leg and repeat. Make sure you do the same number of reps on each side.

Scoop Side Reach

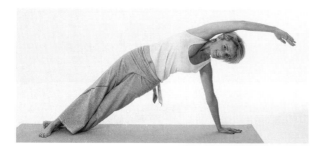

Tip:
Focus on pulling your abs in and up and breathing correctly.

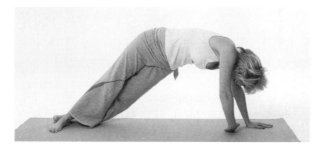

This exercise is also developed from Pilates, and targets the inner and outer waist.

Begin

Sit on the floor, leaning on your left hip, left palm on the floor next to you for balance, right ankle crossed over left, feet on the floor. Lift your body up by pushing off your left hand. Extend your right arm above your head, holding until you find your balance.

Next

Tighten your abs and reach under your body with the right arm. Hold for five seconds. Return to start position.

Do two sets of 8 reps, increasing to three sets of 8–18. Switch to the other side, making sure that you do an equal number on each side.

Rolling Ball

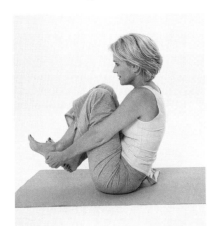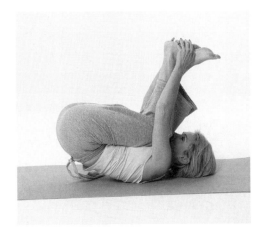

Tip:
Use your tummy muscles to roll back and forth, not momentum. A controlled movement is the key.

This exercise combines Pilates and yoga, and targets the upper and lower abs.

Begin
Sit on the floor. Lean back, curling your spine and shifting your body weight towards the tailbone. Tuck your chin in, lift your feet off floor and grasp the ankles, bringing the heels in towards the buttocks.

Next
Keeping your abs nice and tight and your heels tucked in, roll back slowly and with control until your upper back hits the floor. Hold briefly.

Roll forward without using momentum, keeping your heels tucked in and your feet off the floor. Repeat 8 times.

Side-Lying Kick

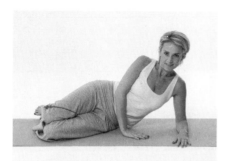

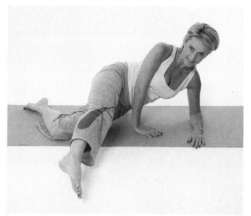

Tip:
Be careful not to lose balance when you kick. Starting in the right position and maintaining muscle control are the keys.

This exercise – developed from kickboxing – targets the outer waist.

Begin

Lie on your left side, supporting your body weight on your left arm with the elbow under your shoulder and bent at 90 degrees. Place your right hand on the floor in front of you for balance. Bend your knees, so your feet are behind you.

Next

Lift your hips off the floor, shifting your lower body weight to your left knee. Keeping the hips off the floor, lift the top leg and kick it straight out with control, foot flexed.

Do two sets of 8 reps, increasing to three sets of 8–18. Repeat on the opposite side, making sure you do the same number of reps on each side.

CHAPTER ELEVEN

Tone Your Tum with Belly Dancing

Belly dancing is one of the most powerful fat-blitzing, muscle-toning ab routines around. It works your abs from top to bottom and side to side. To see how effective it is in making you shapely as well, you only have to look at photos – or even drawings – of belly dancers to see that one of their features is an incurved narrow waist and a firm belly. And you'll burn the same number of calories in a belly dancing class as you would doing a low-impact dance routine – about 200 calories in 30 minutes.

It is a muscle-toning, cardio-intense, low-impact total body workout. It teaches women that they can be strong yet sensual, walk with grace and have a better posture. It keeps the spine and pelvis supple. Researchers at the Mayo Clinic note, 'dancing provides the body with many health benefits. It may help reduce stress, increase energy and improve strength, muscle tone and co-ordination. Dancing can also burn as many calories as walking or riding a bike.' The National Heart, Lung and Blood Institute in the US declared that dancing can lower the risk of coronary heart disease, decreases blood pressure and helps with weight management. It can also help strengthen the bones of your legs and hips. It is also recommended for pregnant women – see pages 97–8.

If belly dancing sounds too exotic and Eastern for you, relax – it's sensuous and exotic all right, but it's becoming far more mainstream in the West. There's even a belly-dancing magazine and if you log on to the various websites you will learn just how popular it's becoming. The US-based DiscoverBellyDance.com is one of the best and contains a wide range of useful articles. For classes in the UK, try the Professional Belly Dance UK site www.bellydance.co.uk which includes, amongst other things, information on classes available in many areas (www.bellydanceuk.co.uk/teacherlistingpage.html).

If you would like a taster, try the following beginner's move. It's great for creating a sexy stomach. If it doesn't inspire you to take up belly dancing, it is still a useful exercise to add to your repertoire.

Figure Eight

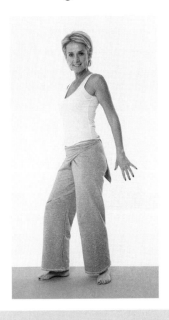 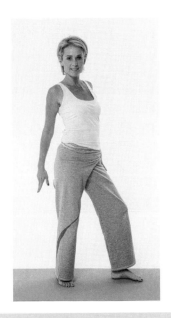

Begin

Stand with your feet flat on the floor, knees slightly bent and arms relaxed at your sides. Start by twisting your right hip forward to make a broad circle outward, then shift your body weight to the left and repeat, making a figure eight with hips and abs, keeping your arms and chest stationary.

Next

Alternate circles as quickly as possible while you suck in your stomach and hold the contraction.

Do this for five minutes a day five or six times a week, for a firmer, sleeker waistline.

CHAPTER TWELVE

Diet – A Crucial Part of the Equation

Let's get one thing straight – if you want to achieve a flat stomach and *keep it*, you will have to watch what you eat. As I mentioned at the start of this book, there's little point having a toned tum if it is hidden under a layer of fat. Now if the very thought of 'watching what you eat' has you reaching for the nearest chocolate bar, think again. It's not about being on a 'diet' for the rest of your life – it's about making healthy eating a part of your life so that it becomes second nature. Okay, so you may have to put some thought into it at the beginning, but once you get to grips with healthy eating and realize just how enjoyable it is – and how great it makes you feel and look – it will be a breeze.

I expect most people who buy this book have a bit of weight to lose but not a vast amount (after all, achieving that perfect flat stomach isn't going to be top of your list of priorities if you have a few stone to lose). As I have said before, the key to losing your flabby tum is to combine your exercise regime with a sensible diet. But what is a sensible diet? These days we are constantly bombarded with claim and counter-claim about the foods we eat and this has undoubtedly resulted in a great deal of confusion. In this section we cut through the hype and provide you with the knowledge you need to improve your diet permanently. And to help you put that knowledge into practice, in the next chapter you will find plenty of suggestions for meals that are healthy, yet low in calories and fat. Now before you flick straight to the recipes, let's look at the all-important knowledge you need to achieve and maintain a flat stomach.

Food is not the enemy

Good food is wonderful – it fuels the body, keeps you satisfied and is a pleasure we can all enjoy. So why is it then that so many people seem to view food as 'the enemy'? Basically, the reason for this is that we have forgotten that the primary role of food is to fuel the body and keep it healthy.

It's hardly surprising really that our view of food has become skewed – for many years we have been subjected to the endless promotion of food as an indicator of wealth, a mood enhancer, a way of saying thank you, a way to keep the kids happy, a way to your man's heart, a means of showing you're cool, a substitute for sex ... Add to this the fact that temptation is under our noses wherever we go, we're living more hectic lives and that everyone else appears to be indulging and you have a recipe for disaster. We're eating more, not because we're hungrier but for social and emotional reasons.

What this basically boils down to is that we are eating for the wrong reasons and we are eating too much of the wrong sorts of foods. Think about it – you don't see fruit and vegetables being advertised as being full of health-giving properties and great for satisfying hunger. No, adverts tempt us to eat fat- and sugar-laden foods such as chocolate – not because they're a good fuel but because they'll make you happy. It's little wonder that food has become such a minefield for so many people. If you want to reach a healthy weight and stay there for life one of the most important lessons you can learn is to use food, not in the way the advertisers would like you to, but in the way nature intended – as a fuel. Eat when you're genuinely hungry and eat the sorts of foods your body needs. By doing this you will actually enjoy your food more and you'll begin to naturally choose all the wonderful foods your body craves – fresh, natural foods that taste great and are full of nutrients. There will, of course, be times when you will feel like a piece of chocolate or some pizza and that's fine – as long as you eat such things in moderation they are not a problem.

So what is a healthy diet?

Having a healthy diet is all about providing the body with what it needs to function properly. This doesn't mean that there are foods that you cannot eat; it simply means that you need to provide your body with the correct balance of foods. So simply increasing your intake of some foods and decreasing your intake of others can make a substantial difference to your diet.

The principal nutrients in the diet are carbohydrate, protein and fat. Carbohydrate should make up the largest percentage of your diet – around 50 per cent, protein should make up about 15 per cent and fats no more than 35 per cent. Let's take a look at each of these categories individually.

Carbohydrates

The carbohydrate category includes fruit, vegetables and processed sugars, as well as starch foods such as bread, pasta, grains and so on. Starches are low in fat, filling and provide energy as well as a wide range of nutrients. However, to get the best out of starchy foods you need to opt for the whole grain variety, not products that have been refined. The reason for this 'refining' carbohydrates such as brown rice and whole wheat to produce their white counterparts results in most of the nutrients being lost. This not only makes the white product inferior in terms of its nutrient content, but it also strips it of fibre – and fibre is important for maintaining good digestive function and may also help reduce blood cholesterol levels.

Sugar

Although sugar is also classified as a carbohydrate, it should not form a significant part of your diet – in fact, the less you eat the better (this of course means refined sugar and not the natural sugars found in fruit). Sugar causes a rapid increase in blood sugar levels, inducing the pancreas to secrete insulin to counteract the amount of sugar in the bloodstream. Sugar may give us a rush, but the pancreas is so effective at its job that it causes the blood sugar levels to dip rapidly, leading to tiredness, a lack of energy and hunger. This roller-coaster ride of high and low blood sugar levels makes us crave more sweet foods and so the cycle is repeated.

But it is not just sugar that induces this response – refined carbohydrates such as white bread are dealt with by the body in the same way. In contrast, natural, unrefined carbohydrates such as oats raise blood glucose at a slower rate and hence keep blood sugar levels stable for longer.

The release of too much insulin also has very important consequences with regard to fat. Many people seem to be under the misapprehension that fat in the diet is largely the cause of fat on the body, and that sugar has little part to play in the process. However, insulin deals with excess sugar by getting the body to store it as fat. This basically means that if you eat lots of sugary and refined foods your body converts the excess energy into fat.

Fruit and Vegetables

Fruit and vegetables also come under the carbohydrate category. They should form a large part of the diet as they provide a wide range of invaluable nutrients. The recommendation is that we eat *at least* five portions of fruit and vegetables a day – and with good reason. The vitamins and minerals found in fruit and vegetables are vital for good health and disease prevention.

To obtain a good range of nutrients from your diet it is important to eat various kinds of fruit and vegetables. However, scientists have recently pinpointed some vitamins contained in certain fruit and veg that are particularly potent. These are the so-called antioxidant vitamins found in dark green and brightly-coloured fruit and vegetables such as peppers, tomatoes, broccoli, spinach, berries, oranges and so on. Antioxidants are basically thought to prevent or destroy excess free radicals – unstable chemicals that are the by-products of body chemistry. Free radicals are highly destructive and can trigger serious disorders such as cancer and heart disease (scientists have in fact linked them to no less than 200 illnesses).

So as you can see, fruit and veg really should be a major part of your daily diet – not only do they fight disease (as well as the signs of ageing), they are delicious, low-fat, high-quality carbohydrate. Do beware, however, of overcooking your veg – steam it or, for the best nutrient content, eat it raw in a salad occasionally. And don't forget frozen produce – it can be just as nutritious as fresh and is wonderfully convenient.

Protein

Protein is vital for our health as it makes up every cell in the body and is therefore essential for growth, tissue repair and maintenance. Sources of protein include meat, fish, poultry, dairy products, pulses and lentils. From a health point of view it is important not to rely on protein sources that are high in saturated fat, so red meats and fatty dairy produce should be eaten in moderation. Lean cuts of poultry, fish, pulses and lentils are all excellent sources of protein. Recently, protein has been getting a lot of good publicity with regard to weight loss but do not be tempted by the trend towards high-protein diets – you will probably lose weight on such a diet but you will undoubtedly overwork your kidneys (as well as experience the joys of bad breath and constipation!).

Many people are unaware that grains, nuts, vegetables and even some fruits supply varying degrees of protein, so the average healthy diet is unlikely to be lacking in protein – particularly if you consider that the recommended daily intake is around 56–99g (2–3½oz). If you're vegetarian, don't make the mistake of relying heavily on dairy produce; it may be high in protein but much of it is also high in fat. Instead, do what so many cultures around the world do and mix your sources of vegetable proteins – have lentils with rice, pasta with beans and so on.

Fats

In recent years, fats have come to be seen as bad for our health. Yet while there is little doubt that our total fat intake is too high – it makes up around 40 per cent of our diet rather than the recommended 30–35 per cent – the widely-held belief that all fat is bad is wrong. Our bodies require certain types of fat to perform various essential functions in the body. We therefore need to look at the kind of fat we are eating as well as our total intake.

Fats basically consist of three types of fatty acids: saturated, polyunsaturated and monounsaturated. Each of these fats provides 9 calories per gram (protein and carbohydrates, incidentally, have only 4 calories per gram) and hence all foods that are high in fat are high in calories. However, each type of fat has different health properties.

Saturated fatty acids are mainly found in animal fats – for instance, meat, milk, cheese, eggs, butter and lard. Saturated fats are non-essential and should be kept to a minimum as they raise the level of cholesterol in the blood and are therefore associated with arteriosclerosis and heart disease.

Polyunsaturates, unlike saturates, are essential as the body needs them to function normally. Polyunsaturates are divided into two groups – the omega-3 and omega-6 essential fatty acids. Omega-3 fatty acids help prevent heart disease and maintain healthy joints, and are mainly found in oily fish such as salmon, sardines, mackerel and trout. Omega-6 essential fatty acids are involved in regulating important body functions – for instance lowering blood pressure and helping stabilize blood sugar levels – and are found mainly in plant seed oils such as pumpkin, sunflower, safflower, sesame and corn. Although the polyunsaturated fats are considered the most biologically beneficial of the fats, processing damages their delicate structure and hence reduces their benefits – for this reason it is best to avoid heating polyunsaturated oils and instead use monounsaturated fats for cooking.

Monounsaturates are found in olive oil, rapeseed oil, avocados and some nuts and nut oils. It is thought that monounsaturated fats may help lower so-called 'bad' cholesterol in the blood. Monounsaturated fats are more stable than polyunsaturates and are therefore more suited for use in cooking.

A word of warning

Watch out for 'hydrogenized' vegetable oils – these have been subjected to a chemical process that changes their structure from polyunsaturated fatty acids to saturated fatty acids. Similarly, when a vegetable oil is converted into a margarine – a process known as hydrogenation – it becomes a trans fat and trans fats are associated with an increased risk of cancer and heart disease.

There is no doubt that fat is a tricky subject. To improve your diet with regard to fats, take the following steps:

- cut down your overall intake of fat to no more than 35 per cent of your total calorie intake
- cut your intake of saturated fat to no more than 10 per cent of that total
- include oily fish in your diet (flaxseed oil is another good source of omega-3 fatty acids – great for vegetarians)

- use polyunsaturated oils for salad dressings – not for cooking
- use olive oil or rapeseed oil for cooking (rapeseed oil has a blander taste than olive oil and is therefore more suited to certain dishes) and, if you wish, in salad dressings
- avoid oils that have been hydrogenized
- watch out for the word hydrogenated on margarines and spreads – if it says 'hydrogenated' on the label it is not a good source of polyunsaturated fats (regardless of which oil it's made from) and should be used sparingly.

Eat smart

Eating smart relates back to my first point about enjoying food as a fuel and not as something to improve your mood or relieve your boredom etc. If one of the main roles of food is to provide energy for the body, then it makes sense to pro-vide it with that energy when it actually needs it. If you think about when you expend most energy and when you take it in, there is often a mismatch. A typical scenario is that we rush out of the house in the morning having had nothing more than a cup of coffee, only to find that low blood sugar and ravenous hunger over-whelm us by 10.30am. We then often opt for a high-fat or high-sugar snack that will give us an instant lift – then feel guilty at our 'indulgence' and make up for it by having a small lunch.

However, the majority of people need energy in the morning and afternoon when they're working – and should therefore be providing the body with the fuel it needs at breakfast and lunchtime. Instead, many people eat a large dinner in the evening, flop on the sofa all night and then wonder why they have a tendency to lay down fat! If you tend not to feel hungry in the morning, look at what time you're eating your evening meal, how much you're eating and your activity level. If you're eating a lot in the evening and you're not doing much, you're probably supplying your body with extra calories it doesn't need. If you provide your body with the fuel it needs when it needs it, you'll be amazed at how much more energy you have.

Watch what you drink

I know everyone's heard it a million times before, but alcohol is full of calories and has no nutrients – so drink it in moderation. Also limit your intake of sugary drinks and those containing caffeine. Sugary and caffeinated drinks result in the same sort of high and lows caused by processed sugars and refined carbohydrates and are often responsible for us reaching for a quick sugar fix when we hit that low.

Instead of relying on sweet drinks and tea and coffee, try instead to keep your water intake up. Many people don't realize it but water makes a great impact on our energy levels. If you're dehydrated – and a great number of us are – you are not providing the right environment for your body to function properly. Water helps our body absorb vital nutrients and flush out waste products. It also swells up the food we eat, making us feel more satisfied. On average, most of us need to drink around two litres of water a day. If you're not used to drinking much water, that may seem like an enormous amount, but increase your intake slowly and make a point of drinking it with your meals and it will soon become second nature. And do be aware that tea, coffee and soft drinks do not count towards your total intake as they actually dehydrate the body. You can, of course, still have a few cups a day – just go easy on it.

One very good habit to get into is to drink a glass of water whenever you feel hungry – often when we think the body is telling us that it is hungry, it is in fact thirsty.

Summary

- Think about what your body needs to fuel itself and stay healthy, and eat when you're hungry – despite what the advertisers say, it's the best reason for eating.
- Where possible, choose unrefined sources of carbohydrate – wholemeal bread, wholewheat pasta, brown rice and so on.
- Cut down your consumption of sugar and sugary products – they cause fluctuating blood sugar levels and can lead to fatigue and a craving for more sugary and fatty foods.
- Eat plenty of fruit and vegetables – at least five portions per day.

- Avoid protein sources that are high in saturated fat – high-fat dairy produce and red meat should be something you have only occasionally; fish, poultry and pulses should be your main sources of protein.
- Reduce your intake of fat in general and switch to healthier sources of fat – monounsaturated fats such as olive oil and rapeseed oil and polyunsaturated fats such as those found in oily fish, seeds and nuts.
- Avoid eating large meals in the evening (unless of course you need them to fuel activity) and instead eat to suit your body's energy requirements.
- Keep your alcohol intake down, avoid sugary drinks and too much caffeine – and drink plenty of water.

CHAPTER THIRTEEN

The Flat Stomach Recipes

This is where we get practical. Now that you've learned some of the basics of healthy eating, this chapter shows you how to put them into practice. There is no doubt that the best way to shape up is through a combination of exercise and diet. If you follow the strategy outlined in the introduction – do your ab routine regularly, take some aerobic exercise every day and eat sensibly – that perfect flat stomach will soon start to emerge. This section is designed to kick-start the process. It provides plenty of ideas for healthy, low-calorie meals that are packed with taste and are surprisingly simple to make.

You can, if you wish, choose a meal from each section and build this up into a weekly or fortnightly plan. This will give you a total of around 1500 calories a day. If you are used to very restrictive diets this may seem quite generous – but remember, you should be doing plenty of exercise so you need an adequate amount of fuel. However, few of us lead the sort of lifestyle that allows us to plan everything we eat to the last detail. If you need to be adaptable (and most of us do) then simply use as many of these ideas as you can manage and for the rest of the time try to opt for whatever healthy, low-calorie choices are available. After all, it's all about making healthy eating work for you, so use these recipes to fit in with your lifestyle.

Breakfasts

Getting a good start to the day is vital. It gives your blood sugar a much-needed boost and prevents that mid-morning energy-crash that can have you reaching for the nearest sugar fix. All the following breakfasts are less than 350 calories. Some are obviously suitable for a chilly winter morning, while others are great summer dishes. A few traditional-style breakfasts in the form of bacon and eggs etc. are also included. Try to vary your breakfast and don't stick to the same thing day in day out – remember, variety is important if you are to obtain all the nutrients your body needs. If you tend not to feel hungry in the mornings and really find it tough to eat breakfast, try the fruit salad or the smoothie – they are not too filling and you'll really notice the difference it makes to your energy levels during the morning. All the following breakfasts serve one.

Great-tasting breakfasts

- Fruit Salad Topped with Yogurt: ½ x 227g (8oz) can pineapple chunks in natural juice (don't forget to add half the juice); 1 kiwi fruit; large handful of grapes; 1 small apple, chopped; 125–150g (4–5oz) tub low-fat natural yogurt

- Porridge with Grated Pear: 30g porridge with added bran, made with water; sprinkle over a little ground cinnamon; grate 1 peeled pear over the top and add 100ml (3½fl oz) semi-skimmed milk

- Toast and Egg: 1 thick slice wholemeal toast; thin scraping low-fat spread; 1 large boiled egg, chopped and mixed with 1 tablespoon fresh parsley; 1 glass unsweetened fruit juice

- Muesli with Blueberries: 50g (2oz) no-added-sugar muesli; 100g (3½oz) fresh blueberries; 150ml (5fl oz) semi-skimmed milk

- Bacon, Mushrooms, Baked Beans and Tomatoes: 2 slices lean back bacon, grilled; 1 large tomato, halved and grilled; 3 large button mushroom, sliced and cooked in a non-stick pan with a few tablespoons of water; 150g (5oz) can baked beans; small glass of unsweetened fruit juice

- Fruit Smoothie: place 100g (3½oz) frozen fruits of the forest in a blender, add ½ x 150g (5oz) tub low-fat natural yogurt, 200ml (7fl oz) skimmed milk (cow's, goat's or soya) and blend

- Cereal and Dried Fruit: 30g (1oz) high-fibre cereal; 150ml (5fl oz) semi-skimmed milk; 3 chopped dates and 3 chopped apricots

- Veggie Sausages, Tomato and Egg: 2 vegetarian sausages, grilled; 2 tomatoes, halved and grilled; 1 poached egg; small glass unsweetened fruit juice

- Stewed Apple with Raisins and Cinnamon: cut 1 large peeled dessert apple into slices and stew in a little water for 5 minutes, remove from pan, stir through 1 tablespoon of raisins, sprinkle over some cinnamon and add 150ml (5fl oz) semi-skimmed milk

- Fruity Bread and Banana: 1 slice fruit bread; scraping of low-fat spread; top with 1 small mashed banana; small glass (200ml/7fl oz) skimmed milk

Snacks

People often find nibbling between meals one of the most difficult urges to control. However, snacking itself is not a problem (most of us now tend to have smaller meals and snack in-between), you simply need to be careful about what you are snacking on. Fruit is great as a snack as it's healthy, delicious and easy to digest. If you need something more substantial, try to opt for a snack that will provide a relatively slow release of energy, such as oatcakes. All the following snacks are under 150 calories. You can have two snacks a day, but try to make one of them fresh fruit.

Simple snacks

- Piece of Fruit: 1 apple, pear, orange, kiwi fruit, handful of grapes etc.

- Oatcake and Cheese: 1 oatcake spread with 1 tablespoon low-fat cheese spread

- Fruit Yogurt: 125g (4oz) tub low-fat fruit yogurt

- Crudités and Dip: 1 carrot and ½ pepper, cut into strips; 1 celery stick; 2 tablespoons virtually fat-free fromage frais mixed with some fresh coriander

- Raisins and Seeds: 2 tablespoons raisins mixed with 1 teaspoon sunflower seeds and 1 teaspoon pumpkin seeds

- Bruschetta: toast a 2cm (¾-inch) slice ciabatta bread, spread with 1 tablespoon tomato purée and top with 1 thin slice fresh parmesan and some fresh basil

- Rice Cake and Peanut Butter: 1 rice cake spread with 1 teaspoon peanut butter

- Dried Fruit: 3 apricots and 3 prunes (the French ones are good) or dates

- Crispbread and Tzatziki: 2 crispbreads spread with 1 tablespoon each tzatziki

- Bagel and Cheese: ½ bagel topped with 2 tablespoons low-fat cottage cheese

Lunches

What we eat for lunch is very much dictated by where we are. Those who work in an office tend to be at the mercy of whatever sandwich bars and shops there are around – unless, of course you take a packed lunch. The idea of a packed lunch may take you back to schooldays but remember, this time you're in control – you choose what goes in it. All the following sandwiches, stuffed pittas and tortillas can be taken to work as packed lunches. Okay so they may take a few minutes to put together in the morning but it means you save time, money and calories at lunchtime.

All the following lunch dishes are easily prepared at home. None of them involve lengthy preparation and all are packed with flavour so don't be tempted to grab any old thing from the fridge. Prepare something for yourself, take some time out and enjoy it. If you're particularly hungry before lunch, have a piece of fruit – it will dampen your appetite as you prepare lunch and prevent you nibbling on something naughty. If you are still hungry after you've eaten lunch, have a piece of fruit. All the following lunches serve one and are under 350 calories.

Sandwiches

- Ham, Mustard Dressing and Salad: mix ½ teaspoon Dijon mustard with 1 tablespoon virtually fat-free fromage frais, spread over 2 slices of thin wholemeal bread and fill with 3 slices (24g/1oz) Black Forest ham, plenty of green salad and sliced full-flavoured tomatoes

- Tuna, Mayo and Watercress: mix 100g (3½oz) can drained tuna in brine with a little finely chopped red onion and 1 tablespoon reduced-calorie mayo; layer between 2 thin slices of wholemeal bread with thinly sliced cucumber and 1 bunch of watercress (stems cut off)

- Mozzarella, Pesto and Fresh Basil: spread 2 teaspoons of pesto over 2 thin slices of wholemeal bread, add a layer (around 30g/1oz) of sliced mozzarella light (use a bread knife to slice it), top with baby spinach leaves and sliced vine tomatoes and squeeze over some fresh lemon juice

Stuffed Pittas

- Artichokes and Blue Cheese: chop 4 canned, drained artichokes hearts into quarters and fry, along with ½ crushed garlic clove, in 1 teaspoon of olive oil. Stuff into a 15cm (6in) wholemeal pitta bread with plenty of strong-flavoured green salad and an individual portion (18g/¾oz) of Stilton, chopped into tiny squares

- Hummus and Coriander: split a 15cm (6in) wholemeal pitta bread and spread with 40g (1½oz) reduced-fat hummus, cover with thinly sliced cucumber and tomato, and ¼ avocado, thinly sliced; stuff in plenty of green salad and fresh coriander and squeeze in a little fresh lemon juice

- Tuna and Sweetcorn: mix 100g (3½oz) can drained tuna in brine with ½ x 195g (7oz) can sweetcorn kernels, mix in 1 tablespoon reduced-fat mayo and stuff into a 15cm (6in) wholemeal pitta bread with plenty of rocket or other strong salad leaf, some sliced spring onion and diced red pepper

Tortilla Wraps

- Salmon and Parsley: mix 105g (4oz) can pink salmon with 2 tablespoons natural low-fat yogurt and 2 tablespoons chopped fresh parsley; spread down the centre of 1 small tortilla wrap, add plenty of green salad, a squeeze of lemon juice and roll up tightly

- Mexican Bean Salad: mix ½ x 300g (10oz) can drained kidney beans with some chopped red pepper, 1 sliced spring onion and 1 tablespoon virtually fat-free fromage frais; spread 1 tablespoon taco sauce over a small tortilla wrap, spoon the bean mixture down the centre, sprinkle over 20g grated reduced-fat Cheddar cheese, add plenty of your favourite lettuce and roll up tightly

- Thai Chicken: mix 100g (3½oz) chopped, cooked chicken breast with 2 tablespoons low-fat natural yogurt, ½ teaspoon Thai red curry paste, 1 tablespoon chopped coriander leaves; spoon onto the tortilla, top with plenty of strong salad leaves and roll up tightly

Some Other Great Lunch Ideas

- Quick Chicken Noodle Soup: simmer 50g (2oz) medium egg noodles, 100g (3½oz) chopped cooked chicken breast and some sliced spring greens in 200ml (7fl oz) vegetable stock until noodles are soft (about 5 minutes) and serve sprinkled with salt-reduced soy sauce

- Carrot, Lentil and Ginger Soup: heat 1 teaspoon grated ginger root in 1 teaspoon olive oil, add 175g (6oz) grated carrot and 300ml (10fl oz) vegetable stock and simmer for 15 minutes; add ¼ x 400g (14oz) can lentils, purée using a hand blender, season with salt and pepper, add 1 chopped spring onion and heat for another 5 minutes. Serve with a slice of wholemeal bread

- Mushroom, Avocado and Kidney Bean Salad: mix ½ x 120g (4oz) bag of your favourite salad leaves with 120g (4oz) sliced button mushrooms cooked in a non-stick pan with a little water, ½ a sliced avocado, ½ x 300g (10oz) can kidney beans and 20g (¾oz) rehydrated sun-dried tomatoes. Squeeze over some lemon juice

- Sardine and Tomato Pasta: fry 1 garlic clove in 1 teaspoon olive oil, add 1 small can sardines in brine, mashed; a squeeze of lemon juice, ½ x 400g (14oz) can of tomatoes and a tablespoon of capers and heat for 5 minutes. Mix through 50g (2oz) cooked wholewheat pasta and serve with watercress

- Baked Sweet Potato with Veggie Filling: 1 medium sweet potato, scrubbed and baked (prick with a fork and microwave on high for 6–8 minutes), then split and filled with ½ x 250g (9oz) pot low-fat cottage cheese mixed with 1 grilled and sliced Quorn vegetarian sausage; serve with salad

Dinners

Many people imagine that healthy eating involves spending hours in the kitchen slaving over a hot stove only to produce something that tastes well, virtuous. If that is your impression, you're in for a surprise – these recipes are simple, quick and packed with flavour.

Each recipe has a serving suggestion – remember, you need to eat at least five portions of fruit and veg a day, so even if there are vegetables in the recipe you should serve plenty more alongside it. This not only provides added vitamins and minerals, it helps fill you up and provides a good ratio of carbohydrate to protein. Do ensure, though, that the vegetables are steamed, lightly simmered or grilled and are not cooked using fats or oils.

Where appropriate, a serving of a starchy carbohydrate is also suggested – but do be careful of portion sizes. Whilst extra vegetables add little in the way of calories (this does not include potatoes, as they are regarded as a starch) and any they do add are far outweighed by their benefits, a serving of rice or pasta can add quite a number of calories. The calorie counts given at the bottom of each recipe do not include the serving suggestion, so look at the calorie count then cook enough rice, pasta or potatoes to take you up to around 550 calories (as I mentioned above do not worry about any calories in the side vegetables). If you fancy a dessert, fruit is the best option. However, if you would occasionally like something a bit more naughty, you can forgo the starchy side dish and use the extra calories to enjoy a small serving of your favourite dessert (just bear in mind those words 'occasionally' and 'small serving').

The choice of dinners is given below, with the appropriate page number for each recipe. All dinners serve two.

- Penne with Broad Beans, Peas and Feta (see page 151)
- Chickpea and Spinach Curry (see page 152)
- Bean, Pepper and Mushroom Stew (see page 153)
- Tofu Stir-Fry (see page 154)
- Salmon and Mango Salad (see page 155)
- Tuna and Dill Fishcakes (see page 156)
- Chilli Prawn and Vegetable Stir-Fry (see page 157)
- Coriander and Lime-Infused Plaice (see page 158)

- Turkey Breast Steaks with Caribbean Salsa (see page 159)
- Easy Chicken Tikka (see page 160)
- Lemon Chicken and Potato Salad (see page 161)
- Spicy Rice with Chicken (see page 162)
- Lamb Meatballs with Yogurt (see page 163)
- Teriyaki Pork with Vegetables (see page 164)
- Mushroom and Beef Bolognese (see page 165)

Nicki Waterman's Flat Stomach Plan

Penne with Broad Beans, Peas and Feta

SERVES 2

100g (3½oz) dried penne, preferably wholewheat
200g (7oz) frozen broad beans
200g(7oz) frozen petit pois
30g (1oz) cubed feta
1 teaspoon fruity olive oil
freshly ground black pepper
handful fresh basil leaves

Place the pasta in a large pan with plenty of water and cook for the time specified on the packet (usually about 10 minutes). When the pasta is half-cooked, add the broad beans and peas and continue simmering until cooked – about 5 minutes. Drain the pasta, beans and peas, place them back in the pan, add the teaspoon of oil and stir well to distribute it. Divide the pasta and bean mixture between the serving plates, crumble the feta over the top, grind over some black pepper and sprinkle with fresh basil leaves.

Serve with plenty of fresh, steamed vegetables – courgettes are particularly nic

Calories per serving: 350   **Fat grams per serving: 8**

Chickpea and Spinach Curry
SERVES 2

1 tablespoon rapeseed oil
1 small onion, finely chopped
1 large garlic clove, crushed
½ teaspoon ready chopped chilli in a jar
1 teaspoon each ground cumin, cardamom and turmeric
400g (14oz) can chickpeas, drained
225ml (8fl oz) vegetable stock
2 tablespoons coconut cream
150g (5oz) frozen spinach, chopped
salt and freshly ground black pepper
½ fresh lemon (optional)

Heat the oil in a large non-stick pan, add the onion and fry gently until softened. Add the garlic and chilli and heat for 2 minutes. Sprinkle the spices over the onion mixture, stir and heat gently for 1 minute. Add the drained chickpeas and the stock, bring to the boil then reduce the heat and simmer for 5 minutes. Add the chopped spinach, stir and continue cooking until the spinach is heated through. Stir in the coconut cream, heat for another 2 minutes, season with salt and pepper and squeeze over a little fresh lemon juice.

Serve with boiled rice and extra vegetables – broccoli is particularly good.

Calories per serving: 310   **Fat grams per serving: 18**

Bean, Pepper and Mushroom Stew

SERVES 2

1 onion, cubed
1 large green pepper, cored and cubed
1 garlic clove, crushed
1 teaspoon chilli powder
1 teaspoon cumin
400g (14oz) can kidney beans, drained
400g (14oz) can chopped tomatoes
60ml (2fl oz) water
200g (7oz) brown cap mushrooms, sliced
salt and freshly ground black pepper
40g (1½oz) reduced-fat strong Cheddar

Place the onion and pepper in a heavy non-stick pan, add a little water and place over a medium heat. Cook, stirring often and adding water when necessary, until beginning to soften. (This is a useful way of cooking onion without the need for oil but it does require you to watch the pan.) Add the garlic and a tablespoon of water and heat for 1 minute. Sprinkle the chilli powder and cumin over the onion mixture, stir and heat for another minute.

Now stir in the drained kidney beans, canned tomatoes, water and mushrooms. Season with salt and pepper and simmer for 15–20 minutes until thickened, stirring occasionally. Divide between the serving plates and grate over the cheese.

Serve with brown rice and plenty of vegetables.

Calories per serving: 278   Fat grams per serving: 6

Tofu Stir-Fry

SERVES 2

1 tablespoon rapeseed oil
1 garlic clove, crushed
85g (3oz) baby corn, halved
1 small red pepper, cored and sliced
85g (3oz) mange tout, trimmed
30g (1oz) water chestnuts, sliced
1 small head broccoli, cut into florets
4 tablespoons soy sauce
1 teaspoon sesame oil
1 teaspoon sherry
140ml (5fl oz) vegetable stock
2 teaspoons cornflour
85g (3oz) beansprouts
2 spring onions, chopped
120g (4oz) pack tofu, cubed

Heat the oil in a frying pan or wok, add the garlic and corn and stir-fry for 1 minute. Stir in the pepper, mange tout, water chestnuts and broccoli and stir-fry for 5 minutes.

Mix the soy sauce, sesame oil, sherry, stock and cornflour together in a small bowl until well blended. Add to the pan and stir until the sauce begins to thicken. Now add the beansprouts, spring onions and tofu and cook for another 3 minutes.

Serve with boiled rice and, if you wish, extra vegetables.

Calories per serving: 295   Fat grams per serving: 16

Salmon and Mango Salad

SERVES 2

2 x 200g (7oz) salmon steaks
½ fresh lemon
1 ripe mango
1 tablespoon fruity olive oil
1 teaspoon balsamic vinegar
2cm (¾in) piece root ginger, grated
salt and freshly ground black pepper
120g (4oz) bag mixed salad leaves

Preheat the grill to medium-high. Rinse the salmon steaks and pat dry. Place the steaks in a shallow ovenproof dish and squeeze over a little lemon juice. Grill the steaks for 6–8 minutes until cooked, turning once and adding a little more lemon juice.

Meanwhile, peel the skin off the mango using a sharp knife, cut the flesh off either side of the central stone and cut into slices. (If you have never chopped up a mango, look out for the large flat stone that runs the length of the fruit. Hold the fruit with the narrowest end upright, place your knife to one side of the tip and gently cut down until you feel the edge of the stone and follow this down. Repeat on the other side.)

Mix together the olive oil, balsamic vinegar, ginger and seasoning. Break the cooked salmon into large chunks. Place the salad leaves in a bowl and add the salmon, dressing and mango slices. Toss gently.

Serve with baby new potatoes.

Calories per serving: 336   Fat grams per serving: 19

Tuna and Dill Fishcakes

SERVES 2

200g (7oz) potatoes, peeled and cut into quarters
15g (1 tablespoon) butter
200g (7oz) can tuna in brine, drained
1 generous tablespoon chopped fresh dill
1 lemon
salt and freshly ground black pepper
1 egg, beaten

Boil the potatoes until soft then mash with the butter. Flake the tuna and add to the potatoes. Add the dill, a good squeeze of lemon juice and some seasoning and mix together well. Add enough of the beaten egg to bind the mixture but don't make it too soft to handle. Shape the mixture into a ball and lift onto a floured board. Now shape it into a large sausage and cut into 2.5cm (1in) cakes. Grill the fishcakes under a high heat for about 8 minutes, turning once, until lightly browned. Prick the fishcakes a few times with a fork and squeeze over the remaining lemon juice.

Serve with a crisp green salad and a low calorie coleslaw.

Calories per serving: 234   **Fat grams per serving: 12**

Chilli Prawn and Vegetable Stir-Fry

SERVES 2

1 tablespoon rapeseed oil

2cm (¾in) piece root ginger, grated

1 garlic clove, crushed

225g (8oz) cooked large or tiger prawns, shelled

1 small red pepper, diced

3–4 spring onions, shredded

Sauce

180ml (6fl oz) chicken stock

1 tablespoon cornflour

4 teaspoons sweet chilli sauce

1 teaspoon sesame oil

1 tablespoon dry sherry or rice wine (optional)

salt and freshly ground black pepper

Heat the oil in a wok or frying pan, add the ginger, garlic, prawns and red pepper and stir-fry over a high heat for 2 minutes. Mix the sauce ingredients together and add to the pan with the spring onions. Cook over a medium heat, stirring constantly, until the sauce is slightly thickened.

Serve with boiled rice or noodles and plenty of steamed oriental greens.

Calories per serving: 334   **Fat grams per serving: 15**

Coriander and Lime-Infused Plaice

SERVES 2

2 plaice fillets, about 150g (5oz) each
1 garlic clove, crushed
2cm (¾in) piece root ginger, grated
3 tablespoons finely chopped coriander leaves
juice of ½ lime
1 tablespoon olive oil
salt and freshly ground black pepper

Preheat the oven to 190°C/375°F/gas mark 5. Remove any dark skin from the fillets (leave the skin on if it is white). Rinse the fish fillets then pat dry. Place the fillets in a shallow, ovenproof dish that is just large enough to hold both of them. Mix the garlic, ginger, coriander, lime juice, olive oil and a small pinch of salt in a small bowl. Spoon the mixture over each fish and grind over plenty of black pepper. Bake in the oven for 15–20 until the fillets are cooked.

Serve with new potatoes or rice and steamed baby vegetables.

Calories per serving: 155   **Fat grams per serving: 10**

Turkey Breast Steaks with Caribbean Salsa

SERVES 2

2 x 100g (3½oz) turkey breast steaks
1 small papaya, peeled and chopped (if unavailable use mango)
½ x 425g (15oz) can crushed pineapple, drained
1 teaspoon lime juice
1 tablespoon chopped coriander leaves

Preheat the grill. Place the turkey steaks on the grill pan, and grill about 10cm (4in) from the heat for 5–6 minutes each side until no longer pink. Meanwhile, mix the remaining ingredients together in a bowl. Serve the turkey steaks topped with the salsa.

Serve with baby new potatoes and plenty of fresh vegetables – French beans and courgettes both suit this dish well.

Calories per serving: 206   **Fat grams per serving: 2**

Easy Chicken Jikka

SERVES 2

150g (5oz) natural low-fat yogurt
1 teaspoon lemon juice
2cm (1in) cube root ginger, grated
½ teaspoon paprika
½ teaspoon coriander
¼ teaspoon freshly ground black pepper
¼ teaspoon cumin
¼ teaspoon turmeric
2 skinless chicken breasts (about 100g each), cut into large chunks
2 tablespoon chopped fresh coriander

Mix the yogurt with the lemon juice, ginger, paprika, coriander, pepper, cumin and turmeric. Add the chicken pieces, stir, cover the dish and set aside to marinate at room temperature for 20–30 minutes, turning occasionally.

Heat the grill to medium. Place the chicken pieces on a foil-lined grill pan and spoon a little of the marinade over each piece. Grill the chicken for about 8–10 minutes, turning and covering with the marinade once more. Sprinkle the chicken with fresh coriander.

Serve with rice and vegetables or a crisp green salad.

Calories per serving: 230   Fat grams per serving: 6

Lemon Chicken and Potato Salad

SERVES 2

juice of 1 lemon
1 tablespoon fruity olive oil
1 garlic clove, crushed
1 teaspoon fresh oregano or ½ teaspoon dried
¼ teaspoon cayenne pepper
2 skinless chicken breasts (about 100g each), cut into strips
450g (1lb) new potatoes
120g (4oz) bag continental salad leaves
Vine tomatoes or cherry tomatoes, cut into quarters or halves
salt and freshly ground black pepper

Mix the lemon juice, olive oil, garlic, oregano and cayenne in a small, shallow ovenproof dish. Add the chicken pieces and set aside to marinate for about 30 minutes at room temperature. Cut any large potatoes in half and boil the potatoes in a pan of boiling water until just cooked. Meanwhile, place the dish with the chicken and marinade under a preheated grill and cook for about 8 minutes, turning occasionally, until the chicken is no longer pink. Add the cooked chicken and any remaining juices to the salad leaves, along with the tomatoes. Cut the cooked potatoes into thick slices and add to salad. Toss the salad, season and serve.

Calories per serving: 478   **Fat grams per serving: 15**

Spicy Rice with Chicken

SERVES 2

100g (3½oz) cooked chicken breast meat
50g (2oz) green beans
1 medium carrot, cut into fine sticks
1 tablespoon oil
1 tablespoon Thai red curry paste
225g (7oz) cooked rice (boiled)
1 tablespoon fish sauce
3 spring onions, shredded

Cut the chicken into thin slices. Steam or simmer the carrot sticks and green beans for 2–3 minutes until just tender. Meanwhile, heat the oil in a wok or non-stick frying pan, add the curry paste and fry for 1–2 minutes. Add the chicken and cooked rice and stir-fry for 5 minutes. Add the carrots and beans and heat, stirring constantly, for another 2 minutes. Stir the fish sauce into the contents of the pan. Sprinkle with the spring onions.

Serve with plenty of vegetables.

Calories per serving: 388   **Fat grams per serving: 17**

Lamb Meatballs with Yogurt

SERVES 2

175g (6oz) lean minced lamb
1 garlic clove, crushed
1 small onion, grated
½ teaspoon chilli powder
1 tsp garam masala
3 tablespoons finely chopped fresh mint
salt and freshly ground black pepper
125g (4oz) tub natural low-fat yogurt

Place the lamb, garlic, onion, chilli powder, garam masala, 2 tablespoons of the mint and the seasoning in a bowl and mix together well until the mixture holds together but is not too soft. Shape the mixture into walnut-sized balls and cook on a grill tray under a high grill for about 8 minutes, turning once. Mix the remaining mint with the yogurt and serve alongside the meatballs.

Serve with a crunchy raw vegetable salad and either baby potatoes or rice.

Calories per serving: 273   Fat grams per serving: 11

Teriyaki Pork with Vegetables

SERVES 2

1 teaspoon oil
1 garlic clove, crushed
2cm (¾in) piece root ginger, finely chopped
200g (7oz) pork fillet, cut into thin strips
1 carrot, cut into thin strips
1 small head broccoli, cut into small florets
1 small red pepper, cored and sliced
1 small courgette, cut into thin strips
3 spring onions, chopped
200g (7oz) pak choi, large leaves cut in half
3 tablespoons soy sauce
2 tablespoons teriyaki sauce
1 tablespoon sesame seeds, toasted (optional)

Heat the oil in a frying pan or wok, add the garlic and ginger, fry for a few seconds then add the pork. Fry for about 3 minutes over medium to high heat. Remove from the pan and keep warm. Add all the vegetables to the pan, and stir-fry, stirring constantly, for about 4 minutes – add a few tablespoons of water if necessary to prevent sticking. Mix the soy sauce and teriyaki sauce together and add to the pan along with the pork and sesame seeds.

Serve immediately, accompanied by rice and green vegetables.

Calories per serving: 308   **Fat grams per serving: 12**

Mushroom and Beef Bolognese

SERVES 2

200g (7oz) lean minced beef
1 garlic clove, crushed
350g (12oz) mushrooms, chopped into very small pieces
400g (14oz) can chopped tomatoes
1 tablespoon tomato puree
1 teaspoon dried basil
1 teaspoon dried oregano
1 teaspoon sugar
salt and freshly ground black pepper
100g (31/2oz) dried wholewheat fusilli
handful of fresh basil

Place the minced beef in a dry frying pan, break up with a fork and cook over a medium heat until the meat is no longer pink. Pour the meat into a sieve to drain away the excess fat. Add the garlic to the pan, along with the drained meat, mushrooms, tomatoes, tomato purée, dried herbs, sugar and seasoning. Stir thoroughly and simmer for about 20 minutes until thickened. Meanwhile, cook the pasta until al dente. When it is cooked, drain and add to the meat and mushroom mixture. Sprinkle plenty of fresh basil over the top.

Serve with fresh vegetables or a green salad.

Calories per serving: 420   **Fat grams per serving: 12**

Index

Banish Back Pain the Pilates Way

Anna Selby, Foreword by Clare Fone M.C.S.P., S.R.P.

Say goodbye to back pain the Pilates way!

Simply follow Anna Selby's safe exercise programme, specially designed for you to perform in the comfort of your home. Not only will this plan help you recover from current back problems but it will also strengthen your back and improve posture so you don't need to suffer from back pain again.

Back pain is on the increase due to modern sedentary lifestyles, stress and the inability to relax properly. Pilates is one of the best forms of exercise to help overcome and prevent back pain – it rehabilitates, relaxes and strengthens the muscles around the spine and abdomen, which support and stabilise the back.

In Banish Back Pain the Pilates Way, Pilates expert Anna Selby has selected specific Pilates exercises that help overcome and prevent back pain and shows you the key areas to focus on. This book also shows you how to avoid a bad back in everyday life, improve your posture to look taller and more confident and strengthen your abdominal muscles to develop a flat stomach.

With *Banish Back Pain the Pilates Way*, you can realign your posture and develop a stronger, healthier back so back pain can become a thing of the past, not of the future.

Juicing for Health

Caroline Wheater

How to use natural juices to boost energy, immunity and wellbeing. Updated with healing Superjuices and the most refreshing smoothies, it's bigger, better and more colourful than before.

Our new edition of this extremely helpful guide to using juice contains all the right updates for today's juice market. Superjuices such as Wheatgrass are now included along with delicious, fresh fruit smoothies.

Juicing For Health includes:
- Over 200 juice recipes and blends.
- The vitamin & mineral content of over 60 different fruit & vegetable juices.
- The basic healing qualities of each fruit and vegetable juice.
- Nutritional therapy juice blends for a whole range of specific – and more general – ailments.
- Beginner-friendly guide to starting up and managing a healthy detox programme.
- A-Z Vitamin & Mineral hotlist – with the "Best Fruits" and "Best Vegetables" for each nutrient.

15-Minute Yoga

Godfrey Devereux

Yoga for a busy world. How to energise and rejuvenate with simple every day yoga techniques.

Fully illustrated with 100 black-and-white photographs, this book is a comprehensive guide to simple 15-minute yoga routines which can be done at any time of the day – essential for busy people with little time to exercise.
As well as introducing the principles of yoga, its benefits and how it works, it also includes:

- Energising Postures
- Grounding Postures
- Opening Postures
- Rejuvenating Postures
- Meditation

These postures will be combined into easy 15 minute practices.
The book also looks at the emotional and physical factors of the practice of yoga – relaxation, sex, pregnancy, diet, fitness, sleep, breath awareness.

Make
www.thorsonselement.com
your online sanctuary

Get online information, inspiration and guidance to help you on the path to physical and spiritual well-being. Drawing on the integrity and vision of our authors and titles, and with health advice, articles, astrology, tarot, a meditation zone, author interviews and events listings, www.thorsonselement.com is a great alternative to help create space and peace in our lives.

So if you've always wondered about practising yoga, following an allergy-free diet, using the tarot or getting a life coach, we can point you in the right direction.

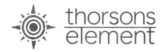